Edgar Cayce
Natural Cures

The Miracle Healing Oil

Called "Palma Christi" - The Hand of Christ

By Sam Sommer

Some Personal Thoughts

Imagine being in the presence of Jesus of Nazareth. What would it be like? How might you react? Is it the same as being in the presence of God? If you were sick, will you be healed? If troubled, would all your worries disappear? Certainly, no one can say for sure, but many have experienced a rebirth just by identifying with Jesus, and those lucky enough to have visited the very ground where he walked and spoke and lived, have told incredible stories of this experience. I received the blessing of visiting the Holy Land some years ago, and to this day, I can tell you exactly what it was like, especially the very moment my plane touched down.

The 747 jet was full of Jews and Christians (as evidenced by their garb) and people of other Faiths and backgrounds. An event occurred at the moment of landing that is difficult to describe, for words cannot adequately capture the feeling. The many hundreds of Pilgrims on the plane started singing, all at the same time. A rush of energy suddenly filled my soul. I knew I had arrived, and what I knew, was that I was home. Home, you ask? I was a 22 year old college student on leave from school for two weeks, who lived in Connecticut. So why did I feel this was my home? Because I felt the presence of my Creator, and I felt that my soul had reached its energy source, the source it had been yearning for my whole life but didn't know it.

It was during my 10 day pilgrimage that I witnessed a series of events, and had first hand experiences that would forever change my life. I saw how people of diverse faiths and beliefs could live in harmony and I found myself changing inside, becoming more understanding and calmer. I realized that God had a plan for me and for the rest of humanity, and it was all good. Toward the end of my stay I met an elderly women who told me an amazing story about an oil that had saved her life and how it worked. She believed that it had been blessed by Jesus and told me to use it when I returned home. So, here it is, the Christ like spirit that I felt in the Holy land, and an oil that actually may contain that spirit.

How was I to know that what she said was true? Could the Christ spirit be contained in an oil? Could Jesus have blessed it? Could it be ministered to the sick and the weak and the troubled? This is the story of "The Palma Christi" or Hand of Christ: how this miracle oil is being used to heal and make souls whole, including my own. May these blessings continue on for you, as they have for me.

- Copyright, Legal Notice and Disclaimer

Introduction

Why is it, that what should be so easy, is often so hard? Why do so many segments of our society lock horns and oppose one another without even doing enough research into an opposing view to determine if there is an element of truth that can form the basis of at least some understanding. This dilemma is exemplified by the medical field. The typical MD is not trained, and in many cases does not have the time or concern to delve into alternative methods of healing, that may relieve the very patients that come for help, and often leave with no more than a piece of paper. On that piece of paper is a prescription for pills that mask or hide the symptoms, but do not cure the disease. Please do not misunderstand me, I am not at all opposed to modern medicine. Emergency care, operations, and many therapies are of great help. I would not hesitate to use this aid when called for. But when people get sick and need to find out why, where do they go? Why don't medical schools research and examine the multitude of therapies that millions of people worldwide take advantage of, and often get relief and cured from?

Here are just some of them:

Homeopathy

Acupuncture

Chiropractic Methods

Massage Therapy

Cranial Work

Flax Oil Treatments

Reams Biological System

Herbal Treatments

Colonic Therapy

Essiac Tea Uses

Hoxey Treatments

Juicing

Vitamin Therapy

Mineral Therapy

Oxygenation

Diet Changes

Fasting

Prayer

Meditation

Exercise

Nucca

Reflexology

I am amused at studies done by Medical Experts and Scientists to prove or should I say disprove alternative therapies. They often do a tiny study and claim: **It Doesn't Work!** It is almost as if they are joyous about the outcome or should I say, they are happy because they can keep getting the big bucks for turn style medicine and paper pushing. After all, if the patient really starting getting better they would not need follow up visits, and the doctor would have to give up the country club membership. Okay, so maybe I am exaggerating for affect, and being unfair. There are many caring and concerned doctors, but unfortunately, here is the bottom line:

We as a people, especially in the United States are getting sicker by the minute. For example, childhood diabetes was very rare just 20-30 years ago, now it is epidemic. Almost 40 % of the population is dangerously overweight. Gall bladders are being taken out in record numbers. People are dying younger, and cancer and heart disease is just as menacing as it was a decade or two ago. No doubt diet plays a key role, but why doesn't the medical field take a stronger stance on issues. Why don't they look into ways of reversing this by using many of the alternatives listed above that can change trends.

Don't believe me? Well maybe you will listen to Dr. Woolf: "There's hardly anything more consequential than Americans dying earlier and being sicker," Dr. Steven Woolf, chair of the Institute of Medicine's and National Research Council's Panel on Understanding Cross-National Health Differences Among High-Income Countries, stated. "That our children are going to die an earlier death than children in other (comparable) countries — I think this is a pretty serious situation. ...On all accounts, humanitarian and economic, this is serious."

Dr Woolf's report that came out in 2013 found that our nation fares worse in nine health domains:

•The U.S. is home to the highest infant mortality rate among high-income countries, and American children are less likely to live to age 5 than children in comparable nations.

•Deaths related to motor vehicle crashes and violence happen at much higher rates in the U.S. and are a leading cause of death for children, adolescents and young adults.

•U.S. adolescents experience the highest rate of pregnancies and are more likely to become infected with a sexually transmitted disease.

•The U.S. has the second-highest HIV infection prevalence among the nations studied and the second highest mortality rate linked to HIV/AIDS after Portugal. The U.S. is also home to the highest incidence of AIDS.

•U.S. residents lose more life years to alcohol and other drugs than people in peer nations.

•The U.S. has the highest obesity rate among high-income countries. Also, beginning at age 20, American adults have the highest prevalence rate of diabetes.

•The U.S. is home to the second-highest death rate from heart disease after Finland among the nations studied.

•When compared to European countries, lung disease is more prevalent and tied to a higher mortality rate in the U.S.

•Older U.S. adults experience a higher prevalence of arthritis and activity limitations than their peers in Europe and Japan.

Almost every major news organization, newspaper, internet blog, and TV station covered this report – in Jan and Feb of 2013.

Look at what happened to former President George W. Bush recently. He looks healthy, has access to the best medical care in the world, is happy, has a lovely supportive wife and family, has no money worries, exercises and has a spiritual connection, yet he could have died had the 95% blocked artery not been discovered via a routine stress test and a stent put in. Medical experts blame heredity and high cholesterol which apparently appeared out of nowhere!

The real story is: How did President Bush get this blocked artery? Does he have a misaligned upper cervical bone? Does he eat fatty foods? Does he chew his food properly? Does he have metal poisoning? Does he have cranial misalignment? Does he lack certain vitamins and minerals? Is he absorbing his nutrients and if not, does he need colonics? Does he drink enough pure water? Does he get enough sleep? Does he go to the bathroom regularly? Does he eat enough fruits and vegetables? And the list goes on.

Why didn't anyone mention these things? The doctors care, but they are just unaware of these options and how they can affect health. I guess the money just isn't there. A heart operation is probably $100,000 or more, while a Nucca adjustment, which could relieve the misaligned bone preventing the signals from getting from the brain to the arteries, cost $75. Or some flax oil therapy which could clear the cholesterol up and only costs $200 - $300.

In this book, and those that follow, we will examine many of these alternative treatments in some detail. Ones that are offbeat, and not widely reviewed, and ones that I have first hand experience with, will be explored. We all live on this earth with common purpose, but until we let go of narrow thinking and egoism, and wealth worship, we will continue to become a less healthy society, and the younger generation now living will indeed stay on track to become sicker that its predecessor.

The "Palma Christi" oil, as an alternative healing treatment, is in a class by itself. This single remedy provides relief and cure to over 300 aliments, and has the record to prove it. For 6000 years it has worked magic. The story of the Palma Christi's history is one of amazement and wonder. Recent scientific studies have uncovered some of the oil's unique properties as they relate to specific ailments, however the fact that this healing agent has benefited so many different types of health complaints over thousands of years, justifies its christening as "The Hand of Christ".

Table Of Contents

Chapter One: What Exactly Is This Miracle Oil?

The oil in question and the plant it comes from has many names. Depending upon what country you live in, and what you use the plant for, it can be called: African Coffee Tree, Castor Bean, Castor Oil Plant, Mexico Weed, Palma Christi, Ricin, Ricin Commun, Tangantangan Oil Plant, Wonder Tree and many others. It is one of the mostly widely known plants, the world over, and has literally thousands of uses: including in manufacturing, the medical field, and as a toxin producer. In fact, the FDA has approved its use in several medical treatments. Every world culture has a name for it because their society has had such wonderful results with it: In Spanish it is called "Aceite de Rcino or Aceite de Castor", in India it is called "Erand Oil", in Arabic it is "Kharwa", in China "Ma Hong Liang", in Indonesia it is "Minyak Jarak".

Scientifically known as *Ricinus communis,* it is a member of the Euphorbiaceae or Spurge family, which has over 300 genera, and over 7,500 species. It is found worldwide: Indo Malaya, South and North America, Africa, the Middle East, and many other regions. It is believed to have its origin in Africa.

For purposes here, it will be referred to as "Palma Christi" or Castor Oil. Castor Oil – Yipes, you say! Okay, so maybe you have used this oil growing up for so called medicinal purposes, but its common use and name is not suggestive of what it can really do, and how it can help you and your loved ones overcome over 300 medical conditions that it has successfully treated. In years past it typically was used as a laxative and taken internally. A newer and now widely known application allows it to be applied on the body heated, with great results. Its benefits have not been fully understood over the years by most professionals, and you and I. When we learn about castor oils God like properties, and how well documented it is as a medical treatment, opinions will quickly change.

Castor oil is made by extracting oil from the castor seed bean. The decorative bean looks like any other bean, but by itself, is deadly. A single bean can kill a child if swallowed, yet the extracted oil can save a life!

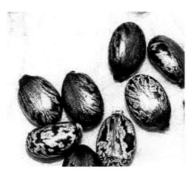

Notice the appearance of each seed – no two are alike

The plant grows to over 40 feet and is not cold hardy. The glossy green leaves are palmate. They resemble the palm of your hand and this in part, suggests, why the name "The Palma Christi" or "Hand of Christ", came into being. The palm like shape of the leaf can at times have ten fingers like your hands do.

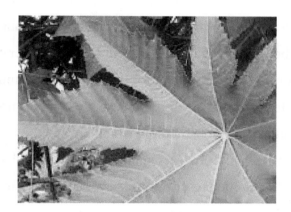

Chapter Two: History of "The Palma Christi" Oil.

Historical records suggest that this oil was in use as far back as 6000 BC. It has been found in Egyptian tombs and was used to fuel lamps because it burns slowly. Its medical and other applications in ancient Egypt, are very well documented, and really quite noteworthy. The plant was sown around houses to repel mosquitoes. Classical authors Diodorus, Strabo and Pliny mention its lamp oil use and that it was used by poorer people to anoint or rub on the body. Herodotus (the ancient Greek traveler), also made note of the fact that castor seed oil was used for lighting lamps and for body ointments, and improving hair growth, and texture. Anointing can mean to rub on or smear on. In this sense it was used on the body as a healing agent. The ancient Egyptian village of Dier el-Medina, which housed the artisans who worked on the tombs in the Valley of the Kings, 3 – 3,500 years ago, used the oil to rub on their bodies to bring relief from the strain of heavy labor. Pharaonic prescriptions show it was used to expel illness in all limbs of a patient, treat head problems, and as an unguent (ointment for burns, rash, skin wounds).

It is said that Cleopatra used it to make her eye whites brighter, vision better, eyelashes longer and thicker. An ancient Egyptian medical document, dating from 1500 BC, describes castor oil as a laxative. As far back as 2000 BC, documents from India suggest it was used in lamps and medicine. These are just a few of many examples of its past applications in many parts of the ancient world.

In ancient Israel, its abundance and ease of harvest made it a great fuel for lamps. This plant seems to spring up everywhere and grows so fast that seeds, loaded with 50% or more of oil, can be taken at will.

While there may be only one Biblical reference to castor oil, it does however reveal an important concept, and historical digging backs this. Here's the complete reference:

Jonah Chapter 4: Verses 1-11

But it displeased Jonah exceedingly, and he was angry.

And he prayed to the LORD and said, " I pray thee LORD, is not this what I said when I was yet in my country? That is why I made haste to flee to Tarshish; for I knew that thou art a gracious God and merciful, slow to anger, and abounding in steadfast love.

Therefore now, O Lord, take my life from me, I beseech thee, for it is better for me to die than to live."

And the LORD said, "Do you do well to be angry?"

Then Jonah went out of the city and sat to the east of the city, and made a booth for himself there. He sat under it in the shade, till he should see what would become of the city.

And the LORD God **appointed a plant**, and made it come up over Jonah, that it might be a shade over his head, **to save him from his discomfort**. So Jonah was exceedingly glad because of the plant.

But when dawn came up the next day, God appointed a worm which attacked the plant, so that it withered.

When the sun rose, God appointed a sultry east wind, and the sun heat upon the head of Jonah so that he was faint; and he asked that he might die, and said, "It is netter for me to die than to live."

But God said to Jonah, "Do you do well to be angry for the plant?" And he said, "I do well to be angry enough to die."

And the LORD said, "You pity the plant, for which you did not labor, nor did you make it grow, **which came into being in a night**, and perished in a night.

And should not I pity Nin'eveh, that great city, in which there are more than a hundred and twenty thousand persons who do not know their right hand from their left, and also much cattle?"

What then do these verses reveal? We know that the Book of Jonah probably dates to the 4th or 5th century before Christ. The Hebrew prophet, Jonah ben Amittai, is sent by God to prophesize the destruction of Nineveh but tries to escape the divine mission. Nineveh was one of the oldest and greatest cities in antiquity. The area was settled as early as 6000 BC but by 3000 BC it had become a religious center for worship of the Assyrian goddess Ishtar. The book of Jonah depicts Nineveh as a wicked city worthy of destruction, hence Jonah's mission from God to preach to them of their coming destruction. After hearing Jonah, they fasted and repented. Because of this God spared the city. Verse 11 states: how they do not know right from wrong (cannot discern between their right hand and their left hand). The book of Jonah, and the rest of the story not mentioned here, is one of the most classic biblical stories.

Now the interesting thing about these Biblical verses as it relates to "The Palma Christi", is the tree that Jonah was shaded under, the tree that sprang up so quickly. Ancient Talmud scholars tell us that this tree in Hebrew is referred to as Kikayon and that witnesses know it as the Ricinus or Castor Oil Tree, and that the sick of the West (Palestine) rest under its branches, just as Jonah did. Note: the Talmud is a complement to the Bible. It fills in the gaps and explains the laws of the Torah (five books of Moses as dictated by God).

The fact that this tree can reach a height of over 30 feet in a very short period helps confirm this

Biblical story: "And the LORD God appointed a plant, ("which came into being in a night") and made it come up over Jonah, that it might be a shade over his head, to save him from his discomfort. So Jonah was exceedingly glad because of the plant." The fact that ancient Jewish scripture refers to this plant as a place for the sick to rest and that God appointed (**appointed can mean decided beforehand and designated**) this plant to save Jonah from his discomfort has far reaching implications.

Dioscorides, the ancient Greek medical scholar wrote a five volume work " De Materia Medica" around 50 AD and in it he describes the Kiki or Castor plant and refers to it as the wonder tree because of its miraculous healing properties. His books are the precursor to all modern pharmacopeias. The story of Jonah is not merely a story of a Hebrew prophet and a tree. This plant is symbolic. Its widespread use in ancient times for light burning oil, healing, and the fact that God appointed it to provide comfort to Jonah and the sick who traveled to Palestine, is not a coincidence. I do not believe that it was by accident that the Kiki plant just happened to be the tree mentioned in this biblical passage. The comfort or shade it brings is symbolic of its healing qualities.

Now the question arises, what is the connection between this plant and Jesus of Nazareth? First let's start with the name - Jesus Christ. The word "Christ" comes from christos, a Greek word meaning "anointed". It is the equivalent of the word *mashiach*, or Messiah, in Hebrew. So, to be the Christ, or Messiah, is to be "the anointed one of God." God anointed Jesus with power – the power of the Holy Spirit and Jesus in turn anointed the sick – healed the sick. He brought faith to many. How did he do this?

What does "anointed" mean? Contrary to common belief is does not only mean pour oil on, but also means: "To smear or rub oil on" (Standard dictionary definition). Jesus was, figuratively speaking, anointed with the Holy Spirit from God. We know that Christ healed the sick and anointing is often referred to in this regard. Some biblical scholars believe that Mary rubbed castor oil on Jesus and that Jesus used castor oil to heal the sick. Rubbing it on - laying on of the hands, may have been what actually happened. This is a logical conclusion because during Christ's lifetime castor oil was readily available, affordable, and was used by the poor. Most other oils were exotic, had to be imported, and were very expensive. Olive oil was available but not used as a healing rub like castor oil was. The poor used castor oil to rub on their tired bodies, so it was likely that Christ may have done this as well.

We cannot dismiss as coincidence the fact that since the middle ages and perhaps earlier, castor oil has been referred to as "The Hand of Christ" or "Palma Christi". It is not happenstance that the Castor plant leaf looks like the palm of your hand and that the oil was used during Christ's lifetime. The fact that it has healed thousands facing medical challenges, and has done this for hundreds of centuries in all parts of the world, is very noteworthy. When we examine the science behind the healing properties of the castor bean oil it will become clear that it is nothing short of miraculous as to how it works, and why it works – it is like a spiritual healing. No other plant has so many uses in such a wide variety of applications, is so easily grown, and found around the world. As we dig deeper into the "Palma Christi" mysteries it will become clear that mere physical healing without the spirit being healed leads to more difficulties. This realization helps demonstrate the Christ like properties of the miracle oil, as it can bring about a spiritual affect. The greatest psychic to have lived, Edgar Cayce, and someone who we will look at in great depth, stated: "There's as much of God in a teaspoonful of castor oil as there is in a prayer!".

Chapter Three: Common Uses of "The Palma Christi" Oil

There are thousands of ways "The Palma Christi" oil is used. Reviewing them helps form a clear picture as to why this product works so well in manufacturing and health. Castor oil is a vegetable byproduct that is odorless, tasteless, and can be clear, or slightly yellow in appearance. The unusual atomic structure of the oil and the ease with which it is derived, allows for a wide variety of applications on so many platforms. Its structure gives it skin absorption viability, allowing the body to take it in so easily. A much more difficult process is needed to transform other oils into practical applications unlike castor oil. As we examine the many uses for it, we come to realize that it is more like a gift to humanity because it can be so easily worked within manufacturing, so easily grown, and most importantly, has so many health benefits that are now just becoming clear to science. The chemical makeup of the oil is of interest.

Average composition of castor seed oil:

Ricinoleic acid 85 to 95%

Oleic acid   2 to 6%

Linoleic acid 1 to 5%

Linolenic acid 0.5 to 1%

Stearic acid 0.5 to 1%

Palmitic acid 0.5 to 1%

Dihydroxystearic acid 0.3 to 0.5%

Note that 85 – 95 % is Ricinoleic acid, which is believed to explain some if its medical benefit. Interestingly, castor oil is the only available source of this byproduct, since it cannot be easily extracted from sclerotium of ergot (A plant which also contains small amounts of Ricinoleic acid). Other listed acids are also of benefit and we will look at them as well.

Over 1,300,000 tons of oil are produced each year, with India being the leader. World production is very large:

India – 830,000 Tons

China -- 210,000 Tons

Brazil – 91,510 Tons

Ethiopia – 15,000 Tons

Paraguay – 12,000 Tons

Thailand – 11,052 Tons

Viet Nam – 5,000 Tons

South Africa – 4,900 Tons

Philippines – 4,500 Tons

Angola – 3,500 Tons

Let's take a look at some of the ways it is put to use. The seed bean is so decorative that it is often used in making jewelry. And what is so amazing is the fact that the genetic makeup of each seed is slightly different – **no two bean seeds look alike. Can you name another bean seed from the same plant where this variation occurs?** The medical benefits are so widespread that a leading Medical Doctor devoted his entire career to its applications because his patients obtained so many remarkable results from it. It is used to make grease lubricants. It is used widely in the polyurethane industry: for coatings, adhesives, sealants, elastomers, flexible and rigid forms. It is part of the building block for Nylons. It is used in a very wide range of pharmaceutical products.

It has unique drying properties when used in paints, epoxy, and coatings.

It is used in a wide range of cosmetics and toiletries and anti dandruff products. Too many to list here. In 2002 it was reported that 971 cosmetic products were made with castor oil in them.

It is used to make synthetic rubber.

It is used to make capacitors and fiber optics in broadband networks.

It is used to make key aroma chemicals in perfumes and many fragrances.

In agriculture it helps preserve feeds, helps grow mushrooms and is used in organic farming. It stops rice, wheat, and pulses from rotting.

It is used to make lamination paper and used to make some inks, especially bio-based inks.

Castor oil has no substitute for its unique biochemical structure. It is made into a unique drying oil that is superior to any other vegetable oil. It is so unique that it cannot be substituted, and it is bio renewable and bio-degradable.

Science has not yet begun to discover its complete industrial potential, and medical science is not even at the threshold of unraveling all of its healing secrets. Do you know of another plant product that has such wide ranging benefits?

Chapter Four: Edgar Cayce and the Miracle Oil

Edgar Cayce (1877 – 1945), often called the sleeping prophet, is perhaps one of the most fascinating people to have lived. The level of his ability to heal through his trance readings and predict the future, has been debated, but the results speak for themselves. Who had a life like his? He was born into very humble surroundings and remained that way until his death, despite the fact that he could have made great sums of money because of his psychic abilities. His 14,306 recorded trance readings on over 10,000 different subjects is, in and of itself, miraculous, especially when you consider much of what he revealed was accurate. He was not educated, and he lived in the pre-techno era. Some report the number of recorded readings is really 14,879 but the figure of 14,306 is what Edgar Cayce's research association lists as accurate. Of these 14,000 plus readings 8,968 had to do with the physical well being of individuals.

His love for and information he revealed about Jesus, has created some of the most fascinating study material ever seen, aside from the Bible. Of these 14,306 recorded readings, the Miracle Oil – Palma Christi, was mentioned 1,390 times. He used it to treat a great range of health challenges with a high rate of success. His large number of recommended uses, and the success it achieved, brought the oil into the public view, and that is why it is so widely known today.

His readings on castor oil point out the fact that merely getting better physically without the soul and spirit being healed, is not the intention. Unless spiritual healing takes place also, the individual will never really be well, since it is the body-mind-spirit relationship that is important, not the body alone. Edgar Cayce suggested that "The Palma Christi" affects the soul, and we will explore this theme. He states that a physical oil can have a vibrational-spiritual affect. There is no doubt that God is at work here.

Information Cayce revealed on healthy eating is considered to be the foundation upon which the health food industry (holistic living) and proper diet is rooted. He spoke about eating an alkaline diet – more fruits and vegetables and less meats (little red meat and no fried foods), before health food stores and the subject of healthy living, were ever born. His 80% raw-alkaline foods program is the gold standard we use today when trying to achieve optimum health. His knowledge of massage therapy, castor oil packs, osteopathic (chiropractic) manipulation, and many other modalities was never spoken of in such depth and accuracy until he came forward with his readings. The information he revealed is considered to be of great importance even today.

President Woodrow Wilson sought the services of Edgar Cayce for healing and guidance while he was President and conceiving the idea of the League of Nations. The prestigious medical journal

JAMA (The Journal of the American Medical Association) considers Edgar Cayce to be the father of holistic medicine.

Recent TV shows that focused on Edgar Cayce, such as those produced by the History Channel, have helped make him more of a household name.

It is vital to have a very good understanding of who he is, where he came from, and what he really tried to do for his fellow man. When you examine Cayce's whole life, what happened to him, what he did for people, and what he is doing today, long after his death, you are faced with a miraculous concept: very few people have had such a positive impact on the physical and spiritual well being of society then and now, and into the future. He is not a God like figure, nor is he a prophet. He never claimed to be. He never took an ego stance and remained a humble, simple person until his death. His work with the "Palma Christi" oil has created the opportunity for millions to be relieved of suffering on so many levels. It is how this oil relates to ones spiritual level or Christ like level, that is important, and is a major theme of this book.

The Edgar Cayce Story:

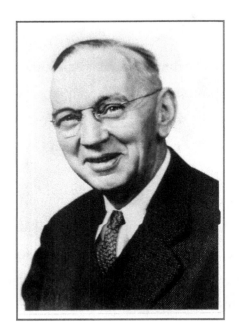

Edgar Cayce In Later Years

Edgar Cayce was born on March 18, 1877 near Hopkinsville, Kentucky. He lived on a farm with his parents, Leslie and Carrie and five siblings. His education was brief, having only completed 7th grade, some say he made it through 8th grade. Even at an early age he began to experience spiritual awakenings and he told his parents he could see angels and speak with the recent dead. He had the ability to sleep with his head on text books and learn the complete book contents and could even quote exact pages and their words. Financial constraints dictated that the young Edgar end school early and seek employment, as was common in those days. He married on June 17, 1903. He and his wife Gertrude Evans had three children.

His psychic abilities became more evident at the age of 21 when he developed a paralysis of the throat muscles and lost his voice. Doctors could not help, so Edgar asked a friend to help him enter a trance like state similar to the one he used to learn text books. His friend gave him suggestions to enter a hypnotic state and while in the trance was able to recommend medication and manipulation techniques that helped him recover his voice completely.

Doctors that lived near Edgar Cayce were so impressed with his abilities that they started giving him only a name and address. He was able to tune in, and figure out exactly what the patient needed to get well. On October 9, 1910 The New York Times carried a two page story about Cayce after a doctor submitted a report on his abilities to a research society in Boston. He was referred to as the sleeping prophet after this article was printed.

The following except from an article entitled "The Life of Edgar Cayce" as found in the A.R.E. (Association of Research and Enlightenment – California and Nevada Region) is of particular interest as it shows how remarkable his powers were, and it details one of his first readings, and the positive results achieved:

"Edgar Cayce felt as if he had been placed in a precarious position. On the one hand, this business of readings was very strange to him. He knew nothing about medicine or the diagnosing of illness. On the other hand, he only wanted to live a normal life with a wife and a family. A friend argued that he had a moral obligation if his talent could be helpful to people. Finally, after a great deal of prayer, after talking it over with his family, and after looking to his Bible for guidance, he agreed to continue the experiments under two conditions: the first was that if he ever suggested anything in the sleep state that could be at all harmful to people, they would stop the readings, and the second was to always remember that Edgar Cayce was first, and foremost, a photographer.

One of the earliest readings was for a five-year-old named Aime Dietrich, who had been seriously ill for three years. At the age of two, after an attack of influenza — which doctors then called the grippe — her mind had stopped developing. Since that time her tiny body had been racked with convulsions. Her mind was nearly a blank and though doctors and specialists had been consulted, she had only gotten worse instead of better.

Cayce put himself to sleep while Layne (A local man, Al Layne, was found to give the suggestions. Layne had educated himself. Not only had he worked with hypnotism, but he was familiar with osteopathy as well.) He conducted the reading and wrote down everything that was said. The sleeping Cayce said that Aime's problem had begun a few days before catching the grippe — she had fallen and injured her spine while getting down from a carriage. The influenza germs had settled in her spine because of the trauma, and the convulsions had begun. The little girl's mother verified the accident. While still sleeping, Edgar Cayce recommended some osteopathic adjustments that were to be carried out by Layne. Layne made the adjustments on the little girl's spine and got a check reading. The sleeping Cayce told Layne he hadn't done them correctly and gave further instructions! After several attempts, Layne was able to carry out the suggestions to the exact specifications of the sleeping photographer. Several days later, Aime recognized a doll she had played with before getting sick and called it by name. As the weeks passed, her mind recognized other things as well, she knew her parents, and finally the convulsions stopped completely. Within three months, Aime's mind was catching up to where it had left off, and she became a normal, healthy, five-year-old girl."

In time Cayce would shift from working to make a living, to giving readings on a full time basis and used donations as a means of support. The demand for his services was so great he felt compelled to follow this path.

The actual way that Edgar Cayce went into his trance like state is of interest. He would lie down on a couch and fold his hands across his chest and breath deeply. When his eyelids began to flutter and his breathing became rhythmical his wife made verbal contact with him. She would make a suggestion to him and Cayce would describe the person in need and give amazing detail about their condition. It was as if he could see into their body. He would then say, "ready for questions" or he would already know the patient's question and proceed to supply information that was of help for that person. Any interruption of this procedure could be dangerous for Cayce and he once remained in a trance state for three days and it was thought he was dead.

During the session, his secretary, Gladys Turner, took notes and recorded everything he said. Cayce was completely aware of what was going on around him as he would often correct his secretaries notes while in the trance if he felt she had not correctly recorded them. Each client was given a number and each reading for that client had the number plus a dash and sub number for each reading. This way they knew who the person was and how many readings were given for that person. So, for example, if they used the number 150 for person X then each reading would be 150-1, 150-2, etc.. Another numbering system was used for group readings and special readings. This way it was clear what the number represented long after the readings were made.

The 14,306 recorded readings contain over 20,000,000 words. Prior to the recorded readings it is believed that over 8000 other readings were revealed, but these did not get transcribed. It is very hard to dismiss as a fake or fraud anyone who reveals over 20,000 documents on over 10,000 subjects when most of the statements were accurate and came true, and are still being used to heal and to predict the future.

The Readings:

Let's look at some of these readings to get a feel for how they are worded, what they say, and how detailed they are. It is extremely important to understand that each reading was given for a specific question, and in many cases the answer was unique to that individual, when the question was focused on a particular person. So for example, if a castor oil pack was suggested for someone, the reading may say to use it a certain way, and for another person who needed the oil packs, their way may be slightly different. This does not mean that unless we use Edgar Cayce's suggestions exactly the right way as it pertains to each individual they will not work for the general population. What it does mean is that we may not have the insight to fully help someone because of a lack of clairvoyance, but we can still apply the remedies, and suggestions based upon the readings, in a logical format. This has worked for millions of people.

To get a sense of the breadth of the readings relating to castor oil, one has only to look inside the health data base housed by the A.R.E. (Association for Research and Enlightenment) founded by Edgar Cayce. Here is a list of just some of them. **(Note: Over 300 Medical Conditions Have Been Treated Using Castor Oil)**

- Alcoholism
- Allergic to Animals
- Allergies
- Animal Bites and Punctures
- Ankle Injury
- Bed Down with Castor Oil
- Bee Sting and Arthritis
- Calcium Deposits and Eye Irritation
- Cancer Pain
- Castor Oil and Allergies
- Castor Oil and Animals
- Castor Oil with Camphorated Oil for Lesions
- Castor Oil's Age-Old Qualities (Facial Neuralgia)
- Childbirth and Castor Oil
- Drug Overdose
- Ear and Nail Problems

- Ear Infection
- Ear Problems
- Fatty Tumor Is Dissolved
- Finger Injury
- Fingers and Eyes and Castor Oil
- Flu, Cysts, Abrasions
- Hair Growth with Castor Oil
- Head Injury
- Hoarseness
- Knee Pain
- Leg Injury
- Minimal Brain Damage
- Nausea, Tumors, Cuts
- Overcoming Wilderness Hazards
- Palpitation and Castor Oil Packs
- Packs for Sprains and Pains
- Packs for the Back
- Pigmented Mole, Lipoma Tumor on Dog, and More!
- Post-Operative Wound Healing
- Pregnancy Stretch Marks, Smashed Finger, Rusty Nail Puncture
- Pterygium, Cysts, Epilepsy, etc.
- Relief from Suffering
- Scleroderma and Polycythemia Vera
- Skin Cancer
- Snoring and Skin Cancer
- Sun and Castor Oil
- Tinnitus
- Tonsillitis and Uterine Infection
- Warts
- Wound Healing

Let's examine some of the castor oil readings and reflect on the information they contain. Most people were helped when they followed Edgar Cayce's advice. All the readings that follow were made by Edgar Cayce in a trance state. The questions are posed by his wife or some other person present. His secretary wrote it all down.

The numbers refer to the numbering system mentioned earlier. This was one of the earliest castor oil readings and the women in question was diagnosed by x-ray as having cancer of the upper bowel:

TEXT OF READING 15-2 Female Age 75

This psychic reading given by Edgar Cayce at his office, 115 West 35th Street, Virginia Beach, Va., this 20th day of September, 1927, in accordance with request made by her son.

PRESENT

Edgar Cayce; Mrs. Cayce, Conductor; Gladys Davis, Steno.

READING

Time of Reading Grand Concourse, 6:30 A. M. Eastern Standard Time. Bronx, New York City.

Now, to meet the needs of the conditions of the body in these changes as have come about are the first conditions to be considered - and these we would keep until there is the change for the better, by this continual reaction for the system, see?

Over those portions of the abdomen where the pressure is seen, where there is the indications of the impacts coming back to the stomach, duodenum, and that portion of the body, we would apply all over, then, this right side those packs alternated between hot saturated solution of Epsom Salts and hot cloths or hot packs of Castor Oil. Keep these continually changing one from the other until there is the relief or the soreness is removed, or the knot has softened, see?

Give those properties as the expediation [expediate - obsolete word meaning expedite] for the system as has been outlined, or as has been used.

For the enemas we would occasionally alternate these in mineral oil or white oil and olive oil, for these will be as foods for the lower portion of the system, as well as active forces for the body. Ready for questions.

(Question) Why has lump in stomach grown from size of a walnut to the size of an apple in one month?
(Answer) Continual packing back in the system. This is a shadow - not a growth at present - from the impactions in the lower portions of the body.

(Question) What is this lump and have physicians with aid of X-Ray properly diagnosed it--one of them saying it is a tumor, the other a cancer?
(Answer) We do not find it EITHER at present - though, with impaction it may become cancerous, or it may take on a tumorous nature, by the natural irritation. At present it is impaction and shadows of feces in the upper portion of the system hardening - that is, the upper portion of the jejunum.

(Question) Have physicians and X-Ray correctly diagnosed this growth as having almost entirely closed passage from stomach to upper bowel and is also gradually closing intestine a little further down?
(Answer) As given here, shadows are the effect of that as seen by the X-Ray. Hence the change in

position and in the condition by change in position of body at time of such X-Ray. True the condition has closed in part the NATURAL tract of the alimentary canal, but with a closed condition would there be regurgitation? or the conditions arising from the stomach as do from continual strain or heaving? By impactions. Do as we have given if we would bring BETTER conditions for this body. Keep these as given - the packs - for this right side of the body of.

(Question) What should be the diet for the body?
(Answer) Little diet will be able to be taken, but that as has been outlined for the system. Those that will be as pre-digested food.

We are through for the present.

What is so amazing about this reading is the fact that the person in question was located in New York and Edgar Cayce in Virginia beach. He saw an impaction, not cancer.

TEXT OF READING 1843-3 Male Age 8

This Psychic Reading given by Edgar Cayce at the David E. Kahn home, 20 Woods Lane, Scarsdale, New York, this 19th day of November, 1940, in accordance with request made by the uncle - Mr. [2413], Associate Member of the Association for Research & Enlightenment, Inc.

P R E S E N T
Edgar Cayce; Gertrude Cayce, Conductor; Gladys Davis, Steno. Mr. [2413] and wife; [337] and [5416] and friends.

R E A D I N G
Letchworth Time of Reading Village, 11:05 to 11:25 A. M. Eastern Standard Time. Thiells, New York

Gertrude Cayce: You will give the physical condition of this body at the present time, with suggestions for further corrective measures; answering the questions, as I ask them:

Edgar Cayce: Now, as we find here, there has not been made - in a consistent manner - those administrations as we have indicted would prove most beneficial in producing the proper coordination between cerebrospinal and sympathetic reactions to the body.

Hence there is not a great deal of change in the reactions in the mental forces as related to physical activities.

In this body, as we have indicated, we find those demonstrations of the necessity of having that correlating, that cooperative activity between the systems of the bodily forces.

We have a very good physical body, but the coordinating of the mental WITH the physical impulses - now - is only existent at times, or periodically.

These disturbances as we find arises from specific conditions, as have been indicated as being a part of this physical manifestation of a body, a mind, a soul, in the material plane.

Then, as we find, those applications that will prove to be the most EFFECTUAL manner of bringing better conditions for this body will be those that will assist nature in breaking up those lesions that prevent this coordination in the present; also to stimulate the nerve plasm to flow more coordinantly through the nerve forces, - both cerebrospinal and sympathetic.

In the present, then, - we would INSIST that these applications at least be given an opportunity to show the effect that may be had upon the mental as well as physical reactions of this body.

The LESIONS exist in those areas of the LACTEALDUCTS" target = "right main" lacteal ducts, or that area just below the jejunum, and upon which there is the flow of activity from pancreas, spleen and liver to assimilate with that digested - or at the main center. Not that there are not LACTEALDUCTS" target="right main" lacteal ducts through other portions of the system, but the lesions are where the greater network exists through which fats and the alkalines and acids are separated in the system.

Here we would apply, consistently (over this area, you see), the hot Castor Oil Packs. These should extend over this particular spot, which is four fingers from the umbilical or navel center toward the right side - only slightly, very slightly upward from that center. If the hand is laid upon this area it will be found to be cold, in comparison to other areas. Then apply these also, or let them extend also, over the liver area, extending to the caecum area, on the right side. Use at least three thicknesses of flannel saturated with the Oil; not just sprinkled on or poured on, but saturate the flannel with the Castor Oil and apply hot. Not so hot as to make it disturbing to the body, but warm; and then cover same with an oil cloth or the like, you see, to prevent soiling of the bed clothing, then applying an electric pad. Keep the electric pad at a heat that is not too objectionable, but warm enough to produce the absorption of the oil into the skin, you see. Let these remain on for an hour each evening, for eight days in succession. Then leave off eight days, then apply again, and so on in this manner.

Following the Packs the area which has been covered by them may be sponged off with a warm soda water solution, to cleanse same.

Then, each evening following the Packs, massage the whole area with the hands gently - not hard - to assist in breaking the lesions here, that hinder this coordination in the activity of impulse. Also massage the SPINE, afterwards - each evening - with Peanut Oil - all the body will absorb; massaging DOWNWARD.

What is so amazing about this reading is the reference to the body, mind and soul and how this medical condition is affecting their normal performance. So, the application of the castor oil packs, which comprises part of the treatment, is helping to bring about a normalization, which involves the soul. We begin to see a picture of how the packs can have a direct affect on the spiritual, as well as the physical, and how they all relate to one another.

Another reading shows that physical hardships help the soul improve:
(Question) How often should the Castor Oil Packs be given?
(Answer) These should be given at intervals of at least three days, until there is no indication of any adhesion through this area. This can be determined by the pressures upon the area over the lacteal duct and umbilical center where they join just below the gall duct emptying into the system, see? and that upon the nerve center just below to the LEFT side of the end of the spine.

Give these Packs three days in succession, you see; then rest three to five days; then give again for three days in succession; and so on.

(Question) Can anything be done at present to improve the leg, or walking?

(Answer) This as we find must be the result of the general improvement of the whole system. This will be GREATLY improved as applications in general are made for stimulating the circulation.

Do not lose patience with self nor with others. Keep the attitude of helpfulness. Know that conditions that exist, while from the purely material may be trying, they are that needed for thine own - and for [2014]'s - soul development!

TEXT OF READING 3690-1 Female age 11

This Psychic Reading given by Edgar Cayce at the office of the Association, Arctic Crescent, Virginia Beach, Va., this 17th day of February, 1944, in accordance with request made by the mother - Mrs. [3691], new Associate Member of the Association for Research & Enlightenment, Inc.

PRESENT

Edgar Cayce; Gertrude Cayce, Conductor; Gladys Davis, Steno. (Notes read to and transcribed by Jeanette Fitch.)

READING

Time of Reading 11:10 to 11:20 A. M. Eastern War Time. New York.

Gertrude Cayce: You will go over this body carefully, examine it thoroughly, and tell me the conditions you find at the present time; giving the cause of the existing conditions, also suggestions for help and relief of this body; answering the questions, as I ask them:

Edgar Cayce: Yes. Here we find very disturbing conditions. For here we have those conditions both of the mental and karmic nature, as well as the results produced by these in the activities of this body.

Some are prenatal, rather as of the entity as a soul-entity meeting itself. Thus this is not a condition to be shunned or to be put away by those who are responsible. For these are parts of the activity needed in the soul-development of those responsible for this body.

This, as we find, in time and in patience may be eliminated to where there may be normal conditions.

When these cares have been taken, there should be an operation - but not until the body has reached the age of at least sixteen to seventeen years. Then the reproductive glands removed will prevent this accumulation from the lacteal duct areas, and the activity in the area of the 1st and 2nd cervical, where the convulsions cause the contraction in this area to the brain.

But through these periods in the next four to five years, there should be kept periodically the use of the Castor Oil Packs. Do this regularly, an hour a day for at least a whole week out of each month. Apply the Castor Oil Packs over the liver and lacteal duct area for one hour each day for a whole week. The next month do the same thing.

Follow these applications each day with a thorough massage, breaking up the tendency for contraction in the lacteal duct area and the gall duct area, and in the 1st, 2nd, 3rd cervical. Also the coccyx end of the spine should be relaxed, after each of the Oil Packs.

These will keep down these contractions.

And then, when the body is sixteen to seventeen years of age, have certain operations as I indicated.

Do that.

Ready for questions.

(Question) What activities would be good for her?
(Answer) Those in the open a great deal, but never where there is not an attendant.

(Question) Has her illness anything to do with failure on the mother's part?
(Answer) No, but the mother may contribute to the entity's soul-development, as well as to her

own in meeting the problems.

We are though with this reading.

The reading above is incredible. We learn about Karmic forces. Cayce alludes to the mother's shortcomings with regard to her soul, and also mentions that the child has severe issues on this level – soul or mental.

The castor packs and other remedies are suggested. This reading shows the strong link between each soul's relation to one another and how physical improvement via the packs can help correct these mental and karmic issues as they relate to the soul. An operation is suggested when the child reaches 16-17 years of age. This is an unbelievable reading that needs further evaluation.

Now what follows are two very detailed and long readings for a 57 year old male. The first reading was given on July 6th, 1941 when the male was 56 years old. The second given one year later. It appears that very profound disturbances exist within this person. However, there is hope for him and these two readings contain some of the most important information ever given regarding our purpose here on earth, and how our soul and body are interrelated.

TEXT OF READING 2528-1 Male age 56

This Psychic Reading given by Edgar Cayce at the office of the Association, Arctic Crescent, Virginia Beach, Va., this 6th day of July, 1941, in accordance with request made by the self - Mr. [2528], through wife; new Associate Member of the Association for Research & Enlightenment, Inc., recommended by Mrs. [2455].

PRESENT
Edgar Cayce; Gertrude Cayce, Conductor; Gladys Davis, Steno. Mr. [2528] and wife, Mrs. [2794].

READING
Time of Reading 11:20 to 11:45 A. M. Eastern Standard Time. ..., Va.

Gertrude Cayce: You will go over this body carefully, examine it thoroughly, and tell me the

conditions you find at the present time; giving the cause of the existing conditions, also suggestions for help and relief of this body. You will answer the questions, as I ask them:

Edgar Cayce: Yes, we have the body here, [2528].

As we find, there are disturbing conditions that prevent the better physical functioning through the body. These are deep-seated in some directions, and should have had much more consideration before this.

But if there is the consistent and persistent application of those things as we will suggest, we find that a great deal of the disturbances may be removed and there may be a great deal yet accomplished in those directions that have been a part of the entity's purpose in this experience.

Much might be said as respecting this entity's attitude toward life and life's experiences. While some may be condemned by a few, would that there were more with that helpful outlook, that ideal which has prompted the activities of this entity.

Many would benefit by practicing those purposes that have been a part of this entity in its relationships to Creative Forces.

But as for the physical, - that this purpose, this mental and spiritual attitude towards its fellow man may have the greater opportunity for further and even greater functioning in this experience:

These are the conditions as we find them, of which the body should take warning, and the manner in which there may be brought about helpful influences.

First, in the blood supply, - we find indications of those disturbances gradually being built in the organs, that bring constantly an upsetting in the abilities of the body to assimilate properly.

Hence we find that there is a torpidity in the liver that is disturbing the whole CENTRAL blood supply. This is producing a character of impoverishment that may eventually bring a form of cirrhosis of the liver itself with which it would be hard to deal.

This not only affects the functioning of the other organs, as the lower hepatic circulation (the kidneys), but the metabolism and katabolism of the nervous system as related to heart and lungs.

Not that there is organic disturbance in either of these (the heart or the lungs), but sympathetic conditions are producing those reactions that are distressing there; through the high nervous forces of the body, aided and abetted by the physical condition and the natural tendencies of an emotional body, causing impoverishment.

Then, in the nervous system, - we find in the central nervous system there are reflexes from the disturbance in the liver, the gall duct area, and the activity of the pancreas is becoming involved. These naturally produce strain upon all portions of the functioning system; yet we find that these at times are well controlled by the mental activity. Again the body becomes so overtired, physically and mentally, as to produce the feeling at times of almost "giving up".

These are the sources, the natures of the disturbances as we find them here with this body, [2528] we are speaking of.

In going about, then, to meet these, - all of the disturbances, as well as the mental and physical reactions, must be taken into consideration.

While these applications may at times appear to be rather severe, we find that they will be most efficient and efficacious in bringing bettered conditions, - if they will be followed consistently and persistently.

First, we would begin with applying hot Castor Oil Packs for an hour each day for three days in succession out of each week. Apply these over the liver, the gall duct and the caecum area, - or from the lower portion of the ribs on the right side, across the abdomen, almost entirely over, and extending to the lower portion of the groin on the right side. Put these on warm, not hot. Use at least three thicknesses of flannel saturated in the Castor Oil, not just poured on but saturating the flannel and wringing it out of the hot oil. Then apply an electric pad. After the heat has raised, turn to low but keep on for an hour.

Then sponge off the areas, preferably with a little soda water.

After this has been done an hour each day for three days, - then at the end of the third day take internally two tablespoonful of Olive Oil; not a tablespoonful and a half, not one tablespoonful, but TWO tablespoonful of Olive Oil.

Then the same three days of the next week repeat the whole procedure, - the Packs, followed by the Olive Oil at the end of the third day.

The next week do the same. Follow the same procedure three days out of each week for THREE weeks, see?

Then begin with the use of the Radio-Active Appliance each evening when ready to retire, for an hour.

Also begin then with osteopathic adjustments, - having at least eight to ten of these, - with special reference to draining the gall duct area.

Through the periods of taking the Packs, or just after the first and second series, and even after the third, it will be necessary to have some enemas or high colonics to remove the poisons from the system. This will aid in establishing better activities through assimilation.

As for foods, - we should supply plenty of the vitamins that aid in body, blood and nerve building. For a tonic, we would take ADIRON; in the beginning one pellet at the heavier meal, but do not begin this until after the three periods of the Oil Packs are given. Begin with the Adiron rather when the osteopathic adjustments and the Radio-Active Appliance are started.

There is the correct balance of vitamins in Adiron as needed for the body; as well as the necessary elements for blood supplying through foods. These are preferably the DON'TS:

Do not take fried foods. All of the vegetables should be cooked in their OWN juices, and NOT with fats.

The meats should consist principally of fish, fowl and lamb, but never ANY of these fried.

DO NOT take carbonated waters, nor any drinks made or combined with same, - especially through those periods that the Oil Packs are given or the osteopathic adjustments - when the gall duct and the area is stimulated to activity.

Begin early in the diet to add especially Jerusalem Artichoke to one meal about once a week. This carries sufficient of the insulin to stimulate the activity between the pancreas and liver secretions, and the kidneys, so as to reduce the heaviness that occurs at times across the small of the back, and the periods when the whole of the outer skin feels as if pulsating - or as if there are the pumping motions through the body.

Do these. Be consistent, be persistent, and we will bring the bettered conditions for this body.

In the mental attitude, the mental and spiritual purposes, hold fast to thy faith in man and God. These are a part of thine own experience.

Ready for questions.

(Question) Who would you suggest to make the osteopathic adjustments?
(Answer) Anyone who is in sympathy with the suggestions indicated. For, these will be found to be the disturbances. DO NOT give this body electrical treatments that are of ANY form outside the body, see?

We are through for the present.

TEXT OF READING 2528-2 Male age 57

This Psychic Reading given by Edgar Cayce at the office of the Association, Arctic Crescent, Virginia

Beach, Va., this 5th day of July, 1942, in accordance with request made by the self - Mr. [2528],
Associate Member of the Association for Research & Enlightenment, Inc.

PRESENT

Edgar Cayce; Gertrude Cayce, Conductor; Gladys Davis, Steno. Mr. [2528] and wife, Mrs. [2794].

READING

Time of Reading 4:10 to 4:40 P. M. Eastern War Time. ..., Virginia.

Gertrude Cayce: You will have before you the body and inquiring mind of [2528], present in
this room, who seeks information, advice and guidance as to how he may be spiritually,
mentally and bodily healed. Also you will consider the invention on which he has been
working, with the idea of saving lives and money, and helping to end the war. You will advise
if he is on the right track to do this with the radar and propeller idea. If so, whom should
he see to make use of it? After giving the information and guidance needed, you will answer
any other questions that may be asked:

Edgar Cayce: Yes, we have the body, the inquiring mind, [2528], present in this room.

In considering the physical, mental and spiritual relationships, - it would be necessary that the
premises be declared from which any reasoning or application of measures would be taken, that
the body may gain the better concept of the relationships that the mental and the physical bear
with the spiritual forces, in relationship to healing of any nature.

The body finds itself in a material world of three-dimensional proportions. That which
manifests in the mental is from or of a spiritual nature, but the results in the material or physical
manifestation depend upon the spirit with which the activity is prompted.

This is the law, that was begun when it was first indicated, "God said, Let there be light, and there was light." This was not as an activity from the sun, or light as shed from any radial influence, but it was the ability of consciousness coming into growth from the First Cause.

Then, what is the light? Who is the light?

These are indicated as the sources, the way. For, as has been indicated, without Him there was not anything made that was made. He came unto His own, and His own received Him not. He was the word made flesh, yet was rejected of men. This, of course, was because of lack of understanding, lack of conception as to the purposes or ideals.

Thus an individual, as this entity [2528] finds self in disturbances of a material nature that are the outgrowth of misunderstanding and misapplication.

Remember, as has been indicated - and as an individual observes, when observing individual souls about one - there evidently must have been, there are, what may be termed confusions even in creation.

These are the results of confusion of instructions or directions by those influences bringing to bear in peoples' lives or activities the result of mental and spiritual activity. These are called accidents or confusions. These may bring into physical expression those hindrances that find expression in both the mental and the material well-being of an individual, - as in this experience here with this entity.

In meeting such, - these may be met, as indicated, in the light, the way, through those very channels in which those misdirections or misconcepts have occurred.

Healing for the physical body, then, must be first the correct choice of the spiritual import held as the ideal of the individual. For it is returning, of course, to the First Cause, First Principles.

For, there was given to individual souls or entities - as to this entity - the ability to choose, or that light (which is the ability to choose for self) - the WILL; to know self to be one with the whole or the Creative Force, and yet choosing the direction or the spirit, or the purpose, the hope, with which it shall be directed.

These are the premises, then, from and through which the application may be made to self, as for physical, mental and spiritual direction for healing.

There are disturbances in the physical body. This we find, then, as to the body forces, as in this body itself:

Each and every entity, as indicated, finds itself body, mind, soul, - or body, mind, spirit. There are, then, those connections, those areas, those activities in a physical body through which spirit and mind function in the physical being for definite reactions or results in the body. These, as we find, are indicated in glands, centers of nerve reactions.

Thus we have a physical being with a circulation through which the assimilation of body forces is taken, distributed through glandular secretion - or mind; that is not conscious mind, but mind of the soul. For, the body IS the temple of the living God, of light, of life, of hope.

All of these, then, are evidenced in a living human organism.

There are hindrances here.

Those tensions need to be released in the physical forces of the body, in those centers where there are the coordinating forces between the mind and the physical reactions, - which are those centers through which the nerve forces in the sympathetic centers coordinate with the cerebrospinal or the central nervous system; or the spirit and mind system with the physical organism, - 9th dorsal, 4th lumbar, and throughout the cervical areas.

Hydrotherapy and massage will help, not hindering those applications being made, as to aid in coordinating the digestive forces of the activity of the nerves.

But keep away from sedatives!

We would have the hydrotherapy treatments, then; not attempting to make adjustments, but sufficient of heat and water as to relax especially those areas; preferably by a Fume Bath with an equal combination of Witch hazel AND Camphor.

These would be given about once a week, not more often than that.

As to the mental healing, - know first thine own ideal. What is thy ideal? Is the author of thy ideal founded in spirit? Is it the light? Is it the Maker of all that is in the earth, be it perfect or imperfect - according to what man has done with this opportunities? But He in Himself was perfect, an thus becomes the light, the savior, the way, the truth, the life. That is the ideal; not merely in a spiritual sense.

For if that light is that which may control the spirit force in self, and in the choice self may take, does it not also then in the same sense control the results as will be obtained in its materialization in the affairs and the experiences of the individual?

THAT is the ideal, and the source of all healing. For, as has just been indicated, - body, mind, soul or spirit are one, even as Father, Son and Holy Spirit are one. For, they are the materialization of the concept of a three-dimensional individual entity or soul, or consciousness of an entity.

Thus the answer must be in the sources of supply, and in accord with that spirit that maketh a soul, an entity, at-one with the Creative Forces, or the First Cause, or God. THAT makes one whole.

As to the ideals of the entity, and its relationships to the purpose as to save others, - these are in the right direction, yes.

The manners in which it may be given to the proper sources may be only through the efforts of the Vice-President, as we find; if there would be worth or the proper coordinated relationships with the ideas and ideals held by the entity.

As to whether this will have its due consideration, - it is the same principle as in healing, the same principle as in relationships to individuals and things. Know thy ideal, that idea you express in the formation of those things as would help. Know that self is correct, - then leave to Him the part that is the purpose of that to be made, to Him who is life and light; putting it in the proper relationships, yes, just as you would your body in its proper relationship to the mind or spirit of the material conditions.

But do not attempt to do God's work, or hinder same, in His cleansing of a sin-sick world!

Ready for questions.

(Question) Should any special treatment or attention be given to cramps in legs, aches in shoulders, aches in toe joints, ill feeling in stomach, nausea, dizziness, and nerves?

(Answer) These as we find, as indicated, come from the inability of those centers and areas to coordinate. With even the second or third of such hydrotherapy treatments, we find that all of these conditions should disappear - IF THE MIND IS KEPT IN THE PROPER RELATIONSHIP AND BALANCE, to self and things without! Don't worry! And what is it to worry? Why worry when you can pray? For He is the whole, ye are the part - coordinating thy abilities with the whole.

(Question) Should anything else be done to give more physical vigor and mental alertness?
(Answer) If we attune the physical forces with the best conditions in the mental and spiritual ideals, you'll be plenty alert - if you find the time to be it! But don't overdo self. Don't overtax self. Not that you are to become lazy; be good, but be good for something!

(Question) Why is it that, although I believe in the power of the Lord, I am unable to get the desired results from my attempts to rely wholly on Him? Wherein have I failed? Is it lack of faith or lack of works, or both?
 (Answer) Read what has just been indicated here. Do the first things first. Lay the stress on those things that are necessary. Remember, healing - all healing comes from within. Yet there is the healing of the physical, there is the healing of the mental, there is the correct direction from the spirit. Coordinate these and you'll be whole! But to attempt to do a physical healing through the mental conditions is the misdirection of the spirit that prompts same, - the same that brings

about accidents, the same that brings about the eventual separation. For it is LAW. But when the law is coordinated, in spirit, in mind, in body, the entity is capable of fulfilling the purpose for which it enters a material or physical experience.

Do that.

(Question) As to the invention, - how may I get in contact with the Vice-President?

(Answer) Write to him and make an appointment - he will see you! Keep in those ways in which there is the putting of the stress upon that needed, see? not attempting to use spiritual forces in the place of mental attitudes, nor use mental attitudes in the place of material adjustments; but coordinating same one to another. And we will bring the complete healing AND a more perfect coordination in every way.

We are through for the present.

Where does one begin when we take a close look at these two readings? They clearly explain that body, mind and spirit are very closely intertwined and that their proper coordination result in optimal health: Here is that statement again:

THAT is the ideal, and the source of all healing. For, as has just been indicated, - body,   mind, soul or spirit are one, even as Father, Son and Holy Spirit are one. For, they are the materialization of the concept of a three-dimensional individual entity or soul, or consciousness of an entity.

The first reading suggests using the Castor Oil packs along with other treatments.

The person who received these readings apparently has good intentions but has tried to use mental forces to bring about humanity's healing. The question posed in reading two, suggests he has an invention that can end the war.

You will have before you the body and enquiring mind of [2528], present in this room, who seeks information, advice and guidance as to how he may be spiritually, mentally and bodily healed. Also you will consider the invention on which he has been working, with the idea of saving lives and money, and helping to end the war. You will advise if he is on the right track to do this with the radar and propeller idea. If so, whom should he see to make use of it? After giving the information and guidance needed, you will answer any other questions that may be asked:

Edgar Cayce makes it clear that this person has created an inbalance in his soul-body-mind. The exact nature of the problem is not clear, but suggestions help us understand what our role here on earth is (let's look at two of these statements again):

As to whether this will have its due consideration, - it is the same principle as in healing, the same principle as in relationships to individuals and things. Know thy ideal, that idea you express in the formation of those things as would help. Know that self is correct, - then leave to Him (God) the part that is the purpose of that to be made, to Him who is life and light; putting it in the proper relationships, yes, just as you would your body in its proper relationship to the mind or spirit of the material conditions.

But do not attempt to do God's work, or hinder same, in His cleansing of a sin-sick world!

Cayce goes on to say:

IF THE MIND IS KEPT IN THE PROPER RELATIONSHIP AND BALANCE, to self and things without! Don't worry! And what is it to worry? Why worry when you can pray? For He is the whole, ye are the part - coordinating thy abilities with the whole.
It seems that at times we try to solve the worlds problems only to find that we have created are own problems by so doing.
(Question) Why is it that, although I believe in the power of the Lord, I am unable to get the desired results from my attempts to rely wholly on Him? Wherein have I failed? Is it lack of faith or lack of works, or both?
(Answer) Read what has just been indicated here. Do the first things first. Lay the stress on those things that are necessary. Remember, healing - all healing comes from within. Yet there is the healing of the physical, there is the healing of the mental, there is the correct direction

from the spirit. Coordinate these and you'll be whole! But to attempt to do a physical healing through the mental conditions is the misdirection of the spirit that prompts same, - the same that brings about accidents, the same that brings about the eventual separation. For it is LAW. But when the law is coordinated, in spirit, in mind, in body, the entity is capable of fulfilling the purpose for which it enters a material or physical experience.

Here is another interesting reading:

TEXT OF READING 1614-1 Female age 38

This Psychic Reading given by Edgar Cayce at his home on Arctic Crescent, Virginia Beach, Va., this 13th day of June, 1938, in accordance with request made by the self - Miss [1614], new Associate Member of the Association for Research & Enlightenment, Inc., through courtesy and sponsorship fund of Mrs. [489], recommended by Dr. [1613] to Hugh Lynn Cayce at New York meeting on May 24th. Miss [1614] is privileged to contribute to this sponsorship fund, at any time in the future she may desire, in order to sponsor another"s Reading who is unable at the time to take care of the membership fee.

PRESENT

Edgar Cayce; Hugh Lynn Cayce, Conductor; Gladys Davis, Steno.

READING

Time of Reading (Delayed on account of late mail) 12:15 to 12:30 P. M. Eastern Standard Time. New York City. (Physical Suggestion)

Edgar Cayce: Yes, we have the body here, [1614].

Now as we find, while there are physical disturbances which prevent the better normal reactions, in giving the causes and their effects upon the physical body much of that which is a part of the heritage of the mental AND physical must be taken into consideration.

There are the inclinations and tendencies towards a LACK of the influences to prevent

portions of the body becoming rather lacking in sufficient energies to keep the system functioning properly; or there is a character of anemia.

From the physical angle, we find that these continue to bring disturbances; especially in the ducts and glands about the assimilating system. These are in the form or nature more of adhesions, that form in the LIKENESS of scar tissue.

Then, this drainage upon the system - as combined with the adhesions (in the lacteal duct and caecum area) - produces a pressure upon the nervous system that causes those reactions in which the body becomes highly sensitive to all the influences about it.

Hence at times, under stress, the effect of odors, the effect of noises, the effect of activities of individuals become as almost OPPRESSIVE to the body.

The reactions upon the nervous system produce at times periods of over exaltation, as might be termed, or over-nervousness; while at other times they become very depressing, with the inclinations for melancholia; becoming rather jerky; and the desire to be alone - while at other times the desires are just the opposite. Yet to all of these the reactions would be to become inclined rather to pity or to be sorry for self, or to blame self for circumstances or conditions with which the body physically or mentally has little to do.

Now as we find, these conditions may be MATERIALLY aided - as they have been - through suggestion, through care, through applications that would become more of a physical nature.

Then:

About three times a week we would apply heavy Castor Oil Packs over the liver AND the lacteal duct, as well as a portion of the central nervous system - or the umbilicus plexus, especially toward the right side. This would mean three to four thicknesses of flannel soaked in Castor Oil and applied as warm as the body can well stand, though not so hot as to burn the body. Leave these on for an hour to two hours. These as we find will relax the system.

Then with suggestion, with massage - gently given; and ESPECIALLY some corrections, with the massage, in the sacral AND the lower lumbar areas, we will find we may break up these conditions.

As medicinal properties we would add as a tonic the preparation called Codiron; this taken twice each day, and must be kept up for SEVERAL weeks, or until at least a couple of hundred tablets or pellets have been taken.

Each day we would also use the vibrations from the Radio-Active Appliance. This would be taken preferably twice a day, about twenty to thirty minutes each period, morning and evening - the last period being just before retiring, or after getting ready to retire. Circulate the attachments each time about the body in the manners as we have indicated for its use; that is: Mark one anode so it may ALWAYS be the one to attach first: Then:

1st period: Make the first attachment to the right wrist, the last attachment to the left ankle.

2nd period: The first would be to the left wrist, the last to the right ankle.

3rd period: First to the left ankle, last to the right wrist.

4th period (which in this case would be at the end of the second day, you see): First to the right ankle, last to the left wrist.

Thus a circle will have been made of the body; the first attached being the positive, the last the negative. Then commence over again. Continue in this manner for ten days or two weeks, then leave off a few days; then begin again - and so on.

These vibratory forces in the Radio-Active Appliance are only controlled in the body, you see; and are not active unless attached TO the body.

Also we find that the low electrical forces, as of ANY electrical vibrations, would be well for the body.

In the diet, keep to those foods that are body-building, blood-supplying; especially - not too acid, not too alkaline. These as we find would have to be judged rather by the reactions that occur, under the directions of one who may make the applications of the low electrical forces and the massage.

When the Radio-Active Appliance is attached, use such periods as the periods for meditation. In thy own words, yes - but after this manner:

See, feel, use the promises that are thine from the study especially of the 14th, 15th, 16th and 17th of John. Let them be as words to THEE!

Then thy meditation:
"FATHER, GOD! IN THY PROMISES, THROUGH JESUS THE CHRIST, I CLAIM THY PROTECTION, THY LOVE, THY CARE!

"MAKE OF MY BODY THAT THOU SEEST AS THE BETTER CHANNEL, THE BEST CHANNEL AS A SERVICE TO THEE.

"RENEW A RIGHTEOUS SPIRIT WITHIN ME. KEEP MY WAYS DAY BY DAY."

This reading, again, shows a lack of balance and suggests that castor oil packs and other therapies should be used. The Radio Appliance, for example, that is mentioned, was used to balance energy within the system. Like a pre Reiki modality. Reiki without a person, so to speak. Reiki is that Japanese founded energy balancing technique used today for many health challenges. Cayce is more precise in this reading, compared to the last few, when he mentions THE CHRIST as the anointer and the guide for the soul. The castor oil pack, along with "THE CHRIST", work hand in hand, on the road to more complete health.

While the Cayce readings previously sited and quoted, focused on the soul and balance, it did not matter what the medical issue was. The intended goal to be achieved was always the same – body, mind and soul weighted properly together to produce health. If the issue was a bad tooth, and the remedy given had to do with teeth, it was part of the whole picture that Cayce was painting – the spiritual advancement of the person and ultimately, the human race.

Note: The word Reiki is made of two Japanese words - Rei which means "God's Wisdom or the Higher Power" and Ki which is "life force energy". So Reiki is actually "spiritually guided life force energy."

Here is another reading for a tumor, along with other challenges. As stated, over 300 medical conditions were successfully treated when castor oil therapy was suggested and used.

TEXT OF READING 385-1 Female ADULT

This psychic reading given by Edgar Cayce at his home on Arctic Crescent, Va. Beach, Va., this 8th day of August, 1933, in accordance with request made by self - Mrs. [385], on her husband"s Active Membership in the Association for Research & Enlightenment, Inc. [Recommended by her husband, Mr. [359].]

PRESENT

Edgar Cayce; Gertrude Cayce, Conductor; Gladys Davis, Steno. Mildred Davis and L. B. Cayce.

READING

Time of Reading 10:45 to 11:15 A. M. Eastern Standard Time. ..., Tenn. (Physical Suggestion)

Edgar Cayce: Yes, we have the body here, Mrs. [385].

Now, as we find, there are many conditions-physical that disturb the better physical functioning of this body.

These, as we find, are rather of the specific nature, though the reactions are quite diffused as to the manner in which the reactions affect the body; and ofttimes in such conditions may effects be treated rather than the causes.

At times the conditions become quite aggravating, and cause a great deal of distress. At others, for periods of days, the body will feel fairly easy, and feel like the conditions are ready   to pass away. Yet, with some disturbance mentally, or overheating, overeating, or any activity that disturbs the equilibrium, the distresses return.

These, then, are the conditions as we find them with this body, Mrs. [385] we are speaking of:

In the BLOOD SUPPLY we find the circulation disturbed, and the blood pressure irregular; the metabolism so disturbed that there are periods when a fullness about the diaphragm area - and about the heart even at times - makes for uneasiness.

These conditions, these disturbances, as we find, are rather of the reflex nature.

In the NERVOUS SYSTEM do we find the greater cause, and the greater effect, and some specific causes of the disturbances in the body.

In the cerebra-spinal system we find, from the very weight of the body - the character of activities that have been from time to time, and from the accumulations of poisons from the alimentary canal, or toxic forces in the system, centers that have become involved by the accumulations about ganglia and centers, that make for the greater cause of the distresses.

These naturally fall into two characters of affectation; those that affect the circulation, from the solar plexus and the lumbar plexus ganglia; and the sympathetic, from the cardiac plexus that radiates with the gastric plexus.

Hence we have segmentations, or segments, that are close in their relative position in the area of the 3rd, 4th and 5th cervical area, in the 4th and 5th dorsal area, and out of alignment in the 12th dorsal and 4th lumbar plexus.

These produce these conditions in the body:

Oft does the body experience that feeling of being a great deal more tired when awaking from what SHOULD be rest-physical, than when retiring. This is the effect of these areas attempting to adjust themselves to a disturbed circulation, by the position and pressure of the organs in the system to the ganglia along the cerebra-spinal system.

Headaches, tiredness in the lower limbs, across the hips, through the chest at times as of a pressure.

All of these are effects of these disturbances.

We find also that, in those activities of the organs themselves - as the liver, the pancreas, the duodenum, the gastric forces of the stomach proper - ALL become involved.

At other periods the effect is to the kidneys and the organs of the pelvis, when there is too profuse an amount of eliminations from the kidneys or bladder; and at others there is too little elimination.

The disturbances through the whole of the colon area are as of a dilated colon in the ascending, and a portion of the transverse - near to the ascending area or colon.

In the effect of that which is produced by the form of fatty tumor that appears, this is rather of the skin or epidermis nature; yet affects the circulation, to be sure, through the presence of the disturbance and the natural inclinations and feelings of the body.

Hence, through this sympathetic effect there is created rather the tendency for the reactions to be such that at periods the body becomes very depressed in its whole mental state. So oft does there arise periods when there appears little or no cause or reason for attempting to carry on. At others it produces a state or period of great agitation to the mental reaction to others; and the apparent feeling as of no one cares, or no one can do - or will do - that which is proper or right, as to the purposes or ideals of the body.

In meeting the needs of the conditions in the present, as we find, THESE would be the manners in which to set up that within the system where not only recuperative forces may set in, but the resuscitation of vital energies stored in the organs in the reactions of the nerve systems.

This may not be expected to occur all of a sudden, but - as the conditions have been gradually growing, naturally the reactions must be slow, especially at first, in bringing about normalcy, or any condition NEAR normalcy for the body: First we would begin as this:

For fourteen to eighteen days, except Sundays, we would have the chiropractic adjustments of the dorsal, lumbar and the cervical areas - see? Take these treatments every day for at least seven days. Then the next week they may be taken every other day. Then they may be taken every day again for another week, see?

After this treatment - not each day, but after the period of treatments - we would use the violet ray each evening for a period of ten to twelve days, each evening when ready to retire,   over the whole of the cerebra-spinal system, beginning at the base of brain and going to the end of the spine, across the lumbar area and down the sciatic nerves; also to the face and head, see?

During the whole period be mindful of the diet, that there is not an over acid diet, but rather that which tends to make for the easy assimilation of the foods - yet strengthening and nerve and blood building, see?

We would also, during the whole period of the thirty days, take - during that period - at least four high enemas, to relieve the pressure in the colon.

For the tumor, or the thickened tissue, we would massage same gently each day with Castor Oil, just what the body and the tissue around same (of the place, see) will absorb. And after this has been massaged, cover with a gauze and let it remain until it's cleansed, of course, in the bath.

In the general, then, the exercises would be such as to keep as near as possible the attitude of helpfulness to someone about the body, about the associates and neighbors, those attitudes that will make for OPTIMISTIC outlook upon all activities.

And we will find, after the thirty day period, there may be given further instructions. This we would do in the present.

Ready for questions.

(Question) Why is my tongue sore practically all the time?
(Answer) From the poisons and the presence of too much acidity in the whole of the intestinal tract.
Hence the necessity of the use of the enemas to alleviate the poisons from the system, see?

As to the manner in which these enemas would be given:

In the first gallon and a half of water we would use a level teaspoonful of salt and a heaping teaspoonful of baking soda. In the last water that is used, use a tablespoonful of Glyco-

Thymoline to a quart and a half of water.

(Question) Why can't I sleep until after midnight, regardless of the time I retire?
(Answer) The metabolism of the system is so disturbed that it is hard for the nerve forces of the body to relax sufficiently for REST to come.

(Question) Why does the least exertion or worry make me wet with perspiration, winter or summer?
(Answer) The disturbed circulation, and the pressures in those particular areas where the cardiac plexus - or the circulation through the respiratory system - is so easily disturbed.

Hence the adjustments will relieve much of this pressure.

(Question) Should I have my teeth extracted?
(Answer) As we would find, these would require some local attention; but not NECESSARY for the extracting of but few.
Do as we have outlined, and - as we find there will be a gradual but sure improvement for the body. And, in thirty days from the time the treatments begin, we may give further instructions. In applying the violet ray, use the bulb applicator for ten to fifteen minutes.

The readings we looked at in this chapter, help paint a picture, and in this picture Edgar Cayce illustrates that health and harmony are obtainable and that mankind is on a Divine mission. We will come back to Cayce and his readings, but for now, a good foundation has been built. As believable as this is to many, there are those who doubt, and claim: how could an uneducated country boy reveal anything of value?

In the next chapter we will provide proof that what Cayce suggested did work and still works. It is virtually impossible to doubt the results of Dr William A McGarey, an M.D., who practiced for many decades in Phoenix, Arizona, and was considered to be a brilliant medical doctor by his peers. His over 30,000 medical diagnoses and healing, based in part, upon Cayce's work, cannot be challenged.

Chapter Five: A Doctor's Story – Amazing Results

Dr William McGarey's story is quite unique. Rather than following the norm, he decided that his career in medicine should take a different path. In fact, he was probably one of the only physicians (M.D.) to include Edgar Cayce's readings as part of his medical repertoire during the 1950's and in some years beyond that. He received his medical degree from the University of Cincinnati College of Medicine in the 1950's. He started his practice in his home town of Wellsville, Ohio and then worked for a short time as a plight surgeon, before settling in Phoenix, Arizona in 1955. He started working with the Cayce materials in 1957. While the focus of this chapter is on Dr William McGarey, his wife was also a physician and she worked with him for much of her career.

Because Dr William McGarey published his findings on castor oil, the focus remains with him but his wife's major contributions to medicine lends credibility to the arguments in this book, so a short Biography is included. This excerpt comes from Psychology Today (not sure when it was printed).

"89-year old Dr. Gladys Taylor McGarey has been practicing family medicine for 63 years. Known as the "Mother of Holistic Medicine" for her role as co-founder of the American Holistic Medical Association, Dr. McGarey brought integrative medicine to America. She's internationally known for her pioneering work in holistic medicine, natural birthing, and the physician-patient partnership.

She was among the first to bring fathers into the delivery room. She and her former husband were the first to bring acupuncture to America and routinely use it in their practices. She began a grassroots movement in 2009 to create a paradigm shift in medical care that promotes the feminine face of medicine. She has been active in the national healthcare movement and continues to visit Washington to educate policy makers why healthcare reform must go beyond payment reform and embrace service delivery reform as well.

Three years ago, riding a donkey at the age of 85, she led a team of doctors into war-torn rural Afghanistan to teach safe birthing practices to impoverished women. This highly successful program has resulted in a 46% drop in the infant/child mortality rate.

She is the author of three books: *The Physician Within You, Born to Heal,* and *Living Medicine.* Dr. Gladys lectures, writes and consults one day a week at her Scottsdale, AZ office.

In 1989, Dr. McGarey founded The Gladys Taylor McGarey Medical Foundation to promote physician training, patient awareness, and practices for personal health that encompass the whole person -- including spiritual, emotional and physical health. Today, its work continues in the U.S teaching doctors, encouraging conscious birthing, empowering women, promoting health and wholeness through education, and advocating for healthcare reform."

After settling in the Phoenix area, Dr William McGarey got wind of a lecture that was being given by Hugh Lynn Cayce, Edgar Cayce's oldest son. The lecture detailed Edgar Cayce's abilities to trance quote information on medical and other issues and what affect they had on people. After attending the event Dr McGarey's own words best describe its impact:

"That was the beginning of the adventure that was to take me through time and space, in a sense, and demand my time and attention, my thought processes, and my writing and speaking abilities for the rest of my life." (quoted from Page 11, The Oil That Heals)

In 1970, both Dr. McGarey's founded the A.R.E. Clinic in Phoenix, Arizona (The name A.R.E. is used through a covenant agreement with the A.R.E. - Association for Research and Enlightenment in Virginia Beach founded by Edgar Cayce in 1931). During its peak the clinic had 50 employees and used a number of Cayce modalities, with emphasis on the use of castor oil packs. The clinic no longer exists but published results by Dr McGarey will serve as the basis for the rest of this chapter.

Dr. McGarey's work established a foundation and reference point so future generations can study the affects of the oil and how it can be used, without fear of ridicule. Not only did he prove, beyond any doubt, that castor oil packs work, but he also demonstrated that they work on such a wide variety of medical challenges that it has no equal when put head to head with any other remedy.

His own words help define and support our objective when he told why he was presenting his findings for all to see:

My objectives, then, are as follows: 1) To stimulate interest in this therapeutic regime; 2) To show the exceptionally wide latitude of use that is possible with the castor oil packs; 3) To present and coordinate evidence that there is actual beneficial response in the human body to the application of these pack; 4) To discuss theoretical considerations relative to the action of the packs on the body; and 5) To begin to explore the validity of a unique understanding of physiological functioning of the human body, which is found in the Edgar Cayce readings.

His case studies and practical experience showed that castor oil has more than a physical affect on the body. It goes very deep and may even reach the spirit or soul, which is part of our makeup, but is generally left to religion and therapy to aid. Let's look at some of his case studies to get a feel for the remarkable benefits of the "Palma Christi" oil.

Dr. McGarey tells us about a man who suffered from inguinal hernia, which usually does not clear up without surgery. At the age of 71 he began wearing a support piece. First on one side, then the other. These went on for six years. Finally, out of desperation he started to massage the areas in question with castor oil. He made over 1000 rotary strokes as he massaged the oil in. In several weeks both sides felt better. He no longer needed the belt. After using this treatment for over a year his condition completely cleared up. Because he kept feeling better he kept doing it, even though a year seems like a long time. He was able to lift a 100 pounds when he felt completely well, a feat that would never have been possible, even if he had an operation. (As reported in the Oil That Heals – Page 23)

In 1967, Dr McGarey, presented 81 cases for readers to review in the A.R.E. March Journal. The following is a recap for some of them that responded to castor oil packs:

Case No. 8.

A 33 year old male accountant had suffered from constipation since childhood. Examination showed no apparent reason but according to Dr. McGarey liver and gall bladder or pancreatic malfunction may account for it. Treatment consisted only of castor oil packs in association with a low-fat diet. The patient cooperated well in applying the packs three days in a row each week, for one hour each time, for a total of seven weeks. Results were very satisfactory. The bowel movements became regular, once daily. The cramps disappeared, and the abdominal pain ceased. Examination showed a normal abdomen with no tenderness elicited. Response rated as excellent to single therapy.

Case No. 13.

A 75 year old was seen for a furuncle (infection of a hair follicle) in the left axilla. She had been hospitalized for the condition many times. She was in tremendous pain and could not move her arm well. Castor oil packs were used twice daily for 1 ½ hours for 17 days. The tenderness and pain subsided within 2-3 days and the furuncle disappeared completely. No external drainage was observed at any time – it just went away.

Case No. 14.

An 11 year old boy was struck by a ball over the right maxilla two weeks prior to being seen by Dr. McGarey. The lump which developed in that area persisted and was growing gradually larger. Examination revealed an 8 mm. fibrous tumor of the subcutaneous tissue overlying the right maxillary prominence, which was tender to palpation. X-rays were negative for fracture. Diagnosis was fibrohematoma of the subcutaneous tissues.

Treatment suggested was use of a castor oil pack to that area for 45 minutes daily, to be used for a period of two weeks. The family cooperated very well, and reported that the tenderness subsided in the first few days, and the size of the nodule gradually became less. When he was examined in two weeks, the tumor was difficult to find because of its size, which was then perhaps two mm. in diameter, and the consistency was softer. Treatment was stopped, and the nodule then disappeared over a period of time.

Case No. 15.

A 37 year old developed a urinary infection three days before being seen on 7/1/65. Symptoms were low back pain and dysuria. His past history revealed two episodes of renal calculus, in 1959 and again in 1963, and occasional upper respiratory infections. Examination showed tenderness over both costovertebral angles, and urinalysis performed on that date showed albumen and the centrifuged specimen to be loaded with white blood cells. The patient was given a sulfa-azo dye medication and the

infection cleared within a week. Infection recurred two days later, but ten days treatment did not now do the job, and the patient was seen on 7/19/65 with original presenting symptoms. Diagnosis was cystitis and pyelo-nephritis. Treatment with castor oil packs was begun on 7/19/65 while continuing the other therapy. They were used over the renal areas of the low back all night long for five days. The aching subsided after the first night, incurred briefly on the third day and then disappeared again. Examination on the fifth day showed absence of tenderness over the left C.V.A., and only minimal tenderness over the right. The medication was cut to half dosage, the packs were continued for another 10 days after that and the patient continued to complete clearing of signs, symptoms and laboratory evidence of infection.

Case No. 18.

An 11 year old schoolboy experienced onset of abdominal pain with low grade fever and vomiting while visiting relatives in California. The physician consulted stated that he had symptoms of appendicitis, gave him an injection of penicillin and advised the parents to go home immediately to seek further care. He was brought to Dr McGarey's office the next day with the history that he had continued to have nausea, anorexia and abdominal pain. His temperature at that point was 98.6 degrees, and examination revealed tenderness in the right lower quadrant with positive rebound tenderness. There was no rigidity, no masses palpable and peristalsis was present. Diagnosis was acute appendicitis.

The mother did not want surgery unless necessary. Since a critical point requiring surgical intervention had not arrived, Dr. McGarey elected to watch and wait, instituting the use of castor oil packs again without the use of the heating pad. The patient was put on bed rest, given only ice chips by mouth, and, with the pack on continuously, he remained comfortable the remainder of that day, He spent a good night, feeling much better in the morning. At that point, his nausea disappeared. On examination, his tenderness was only minimal, and the rebound phenomenon was gone. He was given a full liquid diet, bed test was continued, and the packs were kept on continuously. On the second morning of this therapy, patient was completely asymptomatic. The packs were used two to four hours that day and a light diet was prescribed. Although there were no symptoms and the boy was impatient to be completely active, he was given the packs twice on the third day for one hour each. At that point, his diet was normal and he resumed full activity with no further therapy.

Case No. 30.

A 40 year old married secretary, who was seen with common warts on her right index ringer which had been present for several months. The largest was 8 mm. in diameter.

Diagnosis was verruca vulgaris, right index finger.

These were treated by applying a band-aid to the warts on the finger, the bandage portion being first soaked in castor oil. This was worn continuously, being changed once or twice a day for a period of two months. At the end of that period of time, the warts had completely disappeared.

Dr. McGarey's conclusion regarding the 81 cases will be discussed in another chapter. Here are some more cases he encountered during his many decades of practice.

Horny toe nails are a problem commonly seen among the elderly. It is a difficult condition to correct. Removal does not provide a cure and it is believed to be cause by a fungus. An elderly women with a horny toe nail, large, angled and difficult to trim was instructed to soak her foot in Epsom salt for 15 minutes before going to bed. Then she was instructed to wrap the toe in a small castor oil pack and keep it on all night. She did this for two months. When she was seen by Dr. McGarey at the sixth month mark, her nail was completely normal!

Another unusual case involved a friend of Dr. McGarey. A 12 year old girl had her toes crushed by a man hole cover when it was picked up by some children and then dropped by accident on her toes. After four months of treatment, the toes still had puss and swelling and three orthopedic surgeons were involved over time. Finally, out of desperation, the mother, who had read about castor oil before, poured it in the soaking tub and the toes soaked in it. Several days later they went to their orthopedic surgeon and he exclaimed that "we sure cleaned it up this time". The mother told him, it was not the Epsom salt soaks but the castor oil that did it. While the large toe never grew a nail and remained a bit deformed, the mother was convinced that had they used the oil earlier the nail would have grown in and the toe would be straight.

Hyperactivity is an alarmingly fast growing problem in our society and many attribute it to the diet we have – food dyes, sugar, fast foods, lack of fresh foods, lack of fresh vegetable, etc...It not only affects the young, many older people have this problem. Dr. McGarey had an interesting case involving a young boy with severe symptoms. He was brought to the doctor's office with a belly ache. Three weeks later on the return visit., after using castor oil packs for the belly ache, it was observed that Tommy was sitting quietly and patently on the chair in the doctors office reading. The usual bursts of hyperactivity were not evident.

The story unfolds – each evening Tommy's mother placed the castor oil packs on his stomach while he watched TV (The TV helped him remain quiet). After several days Tommy starting reminding his mother to place the packs on because it "felt so good". He completely recovered from his hyperactivity. In the years that followed Dr. McGarey successfully treated many cases with the packs and good diet. Tommy grew up, got married and brought his kids to Dr. McGarey.

Hearing loss and ear issues often respond favorably to castor oil treatment. One such story involved an eight year boy. He could not hear well out a one ear and had tubes put in twice. His mother revealed that after using the Cayce suggestions, she massaged him, had him do the Cayce head and neck exercises, and used the lamb tallow mixture as suggested by Cayce for four days. She followed this the next evening with a castor oil drop in the bad ear. The next day an amazing event took place. The tube had fallen out and on one side it showed dried blood. His hearing became completely normal.

Snoring is a very serious problem for the sufferer and for those that have to listen to the freight train all night long. Many attribute this to weight gain, jaw position and more. It is often reported that weight loss has many benefits, including cessation from snoring. One couple who used the castor oil packs not only saw the husbands snoring stop but reported that he showed an enhanced sense of humor, more affection, and a spirit of cooperation that just won't quit. If word of this ever got out, the world production of castor oil would fall far short of demand.

Another medical challenge that so many people suffer from, and one that renders the sufferer almost non functional at times, are migraine headaches. I remember my poor dad as he lay in bed day after day in horrible pain and popped Tylenol over and over again. Back then, in the 70's, the alternative options were few and far between and the use of castor oil for other than a laxative, was a closely guarded secret. One case that Dr. McGarey speaks about concerned a 30 year old man who experienced severe migraine headaches since he was 14 years old. All attempts at therapy had failed, just as they had for my dad. But to Edgar Cayce, the challenge was easily met.

Let's look at the whole reading:

TEXT OF READING 5052-1 Male age 30 (U.S. Navy, Carpenter, Roman Catholic) This Psychic Reading given by Edgar Cayce at the office of the Association, Arctic Crescent, Virginia Beach, Va., this 8th day of May, 1944, in accordance with request made by the wife - Mrs. [2466], new Associate Member of the Association for Research & Enlightenment, Inc.

PRESENT

Edgar Cayce; Gertrude Cayce, Conductor; Gladys Davis, Gussie W. Millaway, Stenos. Mr. [5052]"s wife.

READING

(Carpenter's Time of Reading Shop, filing Set bet. 10:30 to 11:30 A.M. Eastern War Time. saws, Camp Bradford, Va.) ..., N.J.

Gertrude Cayce: You will go over this body carefully, examine it thoroughly, and tell me the conditions you find at the present time; giving the cause of the existing conditions, also suggestions for help and relief of this body; answering the questions, as I ask them:

Edgar Cayce: Yes, we have the body here, [5052].

As we find while there are many conditions that are very good, there are those that cause a great deal of disturbance to the body, and become very aggravating at times.

These as we find arise from a condition that exists through the alimentary canal, especially as part of the circulation in the colon. From the pressure there arises the periodic headaches that are the source of the general nervous disturbance in the body.

These as we find may be removed. They are the sources of those that are at times called the types of headaches which refuse to respond to any of the ordinary treatments, and will become constitutional unless there is something done about it.

As we find we would have the application once or twice a week of castor oil packs. If these could be given regularly for several days, it might be more easily eliminated. But when it is practical, at least twice a week, apply over the abdomen, and especially the caecum, and extending up the right side to the gall duct area, castor oil packs. Keep them on for at least one hour or one and one-half hours at the time. Cover this with an electric pad when it has been covered so that it doesn't soil the linens from the oil. Make the pack with two or three thicknesses of flannel, preferably old flannel; saturate the flannel, not just pour on, but saturate the flannel with the castor oil.

The next day taken internally at least 2 tbsp. of olive oil.

Each time following the application of the oil packs, massage the body along the spine, especially the areas from the lumbar axis to that area between the shoulders, with coca butter; massage this thoroughly for at least fifteen to twenty minutes, and let all the coca butter that the body will absorb be rubbed into same.

This as we find, if it is followed, will relieve the sources of this disturbance.

Ready for questions.

(Question) Is this connected with the foot trouble which has recently developed, and what causes this?
(Answer) This is, as has been indicated, a part of the condition. Massage from the lumbar axis. Foot trouble is a reflex pressure on the nerves that lead to the brain through the nerves of the sympathetic system to the cerebrospinal center.

(Question) Should the olive oil be taken the second day of the packs, or after every pack? (Answer) Should be taken after each pack, the next day after the pack is given. Cleanse the portions with a weak solution of soda water, then massage after each pack also. Use cocoa butter in the massage, see? Do that and we will rid the conditions in this body.

We are through with this reading.

The patient followed the suggestions which were given, rather rapidly improved, and later reported that he was completely free of symptoms.

When Dr. McGarey treated women with any sort of pregnancy issue the castor oil pack was recommended. If there were no signs of spontaneous abortion he would instruct his patients to go to bed, elevate their feet and apply the packs without heat. In the majority of cases this technique would allow them to carry to term.

One particular patient has a history of five miscarriages. Each time she reached 2 ½ months spotting would start. She was instructed to stay off her feet and use the castor oil packs in bed as long as she could stand it. If the pack started to bother her, she could take it off. She wore the packs all the way until the baby was born.

She gave birth to two other babies and again spotting started in month three this time and the castor oil packs were used all the way to the birth of her babies.

Another case involving pregnancy, is very interesting. This particular patient started spotting at the six week mark. Dr. McGarey delivered the baby and noticed a perfectly formed harelip scar, all the way down through the soft palate. The patient asked Dr. McGarey when does the lip begin to form in utero and he told her about six weeks, the same time the packs were started. The mother was confidant that the castor oil healed the harelip. Dr McGarey's words sum it up best: "The master surgeon went to work with the Palma Christi and healed that harelip. Therefore, the baby was born with the scar and not a harelip".

Common accidents that appear minor, can often be very painful and can lead to further complication if not treated properly, or if conventional treatment does not do the trick. The castor oil packs have worked wonders with cuts and injuries of this type.

One case involved a 62 year old carpenter with a right index finger injury that occurred 24 hours prior to seeing Dr. McGarey. A large splinter had lodged into the the tissues of the dorsum near the nail. The carpenter got it out prior to the visit. Upon examination it was clear that the tissue was acutely inflamed causing swelling. Dr. McGarey made a small incision and removed a 5/8 inch intact splinter which allowed the injury to drain. Castor oil was applied, surrounded with plastic and gauze for 48 hours. What is so unusual about the case is that upon examination after 2 days, the level of healing was profound and often never seen to occur so quickly in these situations without post operative care.

Another medical difficulty concerned a 17 year female high school senior with pain in the left arm from a physical education class injury. While doing pull ups she suddenly developed a sharp pain and her left forearm started to swell. Examination revealed sprain of the left biceps muscle at its radial intersection.

Treatment consisted of castor oil packs over the entire proximal half of the left forearm and the elbow daily. To be left on all night long and left on as much during the day as possible. Three days later, examination revealed all tenderness to be gone and swelling subsided.

Dr McGarey relates the story of a call from the emergency room for a patient who had sprained her ankle at work. X-rays revealed no fracture, but she had difficulty putting any weight on the foot. It should be noted that injuries like this often take weeks and sometimes months to heal completely. She was instructed to wear a castor oil pack for the next two days using plastic wrap and elastic bandage to hold it in place providing some pressure to help the swelling.

Two days later, she appeared at the office, walking normally with the pack in place. Dr. McGarey relates how she found the treatment to be so strange: "What am I doing? That is the craziest thing I heard of." Since she knew nothing else to do and the ankle was hurting, she followed the instructions.

She used the pack for the next few days walking without a limp and no pain. It was surprising at how fast the positive response was.

Tumors are a frightening thing and when you discover that you have one or more, it becomes very challenging, both physically and mentally. This is especially true for women, as lumps in the breast are constantly mentioned with regard to self checking. One such case for another patient started when a small breast lump was discovered. She started using the castor oil packs for one week as advised, with the resolve that if that did not work she would have it removed surgically.

She proceeded to place an oil pack covered with plastic on her breast and wore it for one whole week under a bra, which she normally does not wear. At the end of the week while sitting at her desk at work she felt a gush of liquid come through her armpit. Thinking it was a cyst, it apparently had burst. Touching the breast revealed that the lump was gone. Ten years later there were no recurrences.

According to Dr. McGarey, appendicitis is a difficult problem both to diagnose and to treat. An 11 year old complained of pain and it appeared to be inflamed appendix. Castor oil packs overnight maintained a state of semi-status quo, His white blood cell count was only 5,300 with 70% polys; and urine showed a few white cells and a trace of albumen. Sixteen hours after onset, acupuncture was accomplished just below stomach point #36, with relief of much of the tenderness. There was no vomiting, but there was a low grade fever of 99.8 degrees. Diet was limited to clear liquids. The parents declined surgery after surgical consultation suggested it be done. At 36 hours after onset another acupuncture was administered. After another night with continued packs, all symptoms were gone by the next morning. The patient resumed his activities with no subsequent problem, and a follow-up blood count was normal.

Dr. McGarey states that this case clearly supports his observations that twelve of thirteen cases of clinically diagnosed appendicitis were cleared up using only castor oil packs, with ice chips and sips of fluid as the only diet.

I have presented a few of Dr. McGarey's castor oil pack success stories to help verify the contention that it can be a healing agent of first choice for a wide variety of illnesses. More of Dr. McGarey's work and opinion will be presented when we look at the theories that try to explain how castor oil works, what it does to the body-mind-soul during recovery from health challenges.

Chapter Six: How Does It Work – The Spiritual Factor?

In trying to understand the science behind "The Palma Christi" we will have to dig deep into the minds of Cayce, McGarey and many others, but in the end we may come up just a little short. While Cayce gave many explanations about the way or how castor oil heals, the greatest minds of today and yesterday (Dr. McGarey, for example), have yet to catch up with his brilliance. He describes parts of the body and physiological relations that are not discussed in medical literature , and may only dwell in the heavens above for some time to come.

Let's look at the chemical composition of castor oil again. Notice how Ricinoleic acid makes up 85% - 95% of the oil and oleic acid 2% - 6%.

Average composition of castor seed oil

Acid name   Average Percentage Range

Ricinoleic acid   85 to 95%

Oleic acid   2 to 6 %

Linoleic acid 1 to 5%

Linolenic acid .5 to 1 %

Stearic acid   0.5 to 1%

Palmitic acid 0.5 to 1%

Dihydroxystearic acid 0.3 to 0.5%

Others 0.2 to 0.5%

In 1961 in the Journal of American Oil Chemists' Society, A.F. Novak writes how ricinoleic and oleic acid derivatives were studied for their antimicrobial properties and found that these two substances were superior in their activity against several species of bacteria, yeasts and molds when compared to sorbic and 10-undecenoic acids, two known antimicrobial agents. This explains why castor oil has been used successfully in treating puncture wounds; even when the patient is experiencing an acute infection at the wound site.

Many studies have been done on castor oil topically and internally:

An Indian study in 2011 found that castor leaf extract showed better antibacterial activity against both Gram-positive and Gram-negative bacteria than Gentamycin (their standard for comparison).

A 2010 study found that castor oil packs were an effective means of decreasing constipation in the elderly.

In 2009 a study found that castor oil effectively relieves arthritis symptoms.

A 1999 study was carried out to determine whether or not topical castor oil would stimulate the lymphatic system. The findings were positive. After a two-hour treatment with castor oil packs, there was a significant increase in the number of T-11 cells, which increased over a seven-hour period following treatment.

In this 2000 study of the effects of ricinoleic acid on inflammation, researchers found it exerted "capsaicin-like" anti inflammatory properties.

Another study states that patients with occupational dermatitis may have a positive reaction to castor oil or ricinoleic acid

These and many other studies suggest that castor oil does work and it works on several levels. It has anti inflammatory properties, anti microbial value, and helps the immune system.

This information is very important as we piece this big puzzle together but we still haven't addressed the issue of how does one remedy work on so many levels and affect the healing process for so many different types of health challenges? It must work on a much deeper level than as an anti inflammatory, anti microbial and immune system helper.

It is important to comment on a term that Cayce uses in his readings and one that will be mentioned in the pages ahead when we quote Dr. McGarey as he attempts to explain how castor oil packs work. Dr. McGarey mentions "Peyer Patches", and gives some explanation, but a more detailed view may help to better understand his upcoming comments.

As found in Wikipedia:

"Peyer's patches (or aggregated lymphoid nodules) are organized lymphoid nodules, named after the 17th-century Swiss anatomist Johann Conrad Peyer. They are aggregations of lymphoid tissue that are usually found in the lowest portion of the small intestine, the ileum, in humans; as such, they differentiate the ileum from the duodenum and jejunum.

Because the lumen of the gastrointestinal tract is exposed to the external environment, much of it is populated with potentially pathogenic microorganisms. Peyer's patches thus establish their importance in the immune surveillance of the intestinal lumen and in facilitating the generation of the immune response within the mucosa."

In other words, if they are working correctly, the immune system is also working correctly. Dr. McGarey found that total lymphocyte count increased significantly when castor oil packs were used and that T-pan lymphocyte count (T-11 cells) also increased. The thymus gland and other component parts of the immune system were also enhanced from the castor oil packs.

Dr. McGarey believed that castor oil may create a vibration within the body that is more easily attuned to Creative Forces and thus bring about healing activity.

Perhaps no one is in a better position to try and get a handle on the miracles of castor oil than Dr. McGarey. His commentary in the A.R.E. Journal, March, 1967, Volume 2, No. 2, page 3 provides one of the best insights into this subject, and as such, it is quoted in its entirety:

These statements that I will now read from Dr. McGarey are interspersed with statements from Cayce.

"How does castor oil as a pack act in the human body? How does it bring into being a beneficial effect in body tissues? Among other things, we observed that the packs, when used in the 81 cases, produced the following results: brought a peaceful sensation to the abdomen; affected beneficially the autonomic; induced changes in the lymphatics; relieved bodily stress; restored curly hair (!); apparently affected ganglia and plexuses; cleared up infections; aided pregnancy; benefited systems (e.g. genito-urinary); and affected beneficially areas of the body such as the pelvic organs.

Cayce, in his readings, gives us ideas relative to the effects that castor oil has in the body when applied in such a manner, but the understanding is not easy to come by. I would like to use two references first, then comment on them. The first was an answer to a question about a psychic experience the woman had, and Cayce brings the castor oil into this discussion, relating it significantly, I think. The second extract is from an earlier reading given the same woman who had been applying psychic information from Cayce for two years, and was highly desirous of becoming pregnant."

Cayce states:

This was an inter-between emotion, or as indicated - a partial psychic experience. Consider that which takes place from the use of the oil pack and its influence upon the body, and something of the emotion experienced may be partially understood.

Oil is that which constitutes, in a form, the nature of activity between the functionings of the organs of the system as related to activity. Much in the same manner as oil would act upon an inanimate object - it acts as a limbering agent, allowing movement, motion, as may be had by the attempt to move a hinge, a wrench, a center, or that movement of an inanimate machinery motion. This is the same effect had upon that which is now animated by spirit. This movement, then, was the reflection of the abilities of the spirit of ANIMATE activity as controlled through the emotions of mind, or the activity of mind between spirit AND matter. This was a vision, see? (1523-14)

Cayce states:

Then, for the betterment of the general conditions as a whole, it would be well that much of an analysis be given; that the conditions which are existent be thoroughly understood from a psychological, pathological and physiological standpoint. These are not meant to be mere terms, but indicate rather the boundaries of the various changes which have taken place, and are taking place, in this body. In other words, then:

The body, as an entity, is experiencing the result of the mental attitudes of the body through a given period. Thus, psychological conditions have brought, do bring, their effect upon the general systems of the body. Hence, these are - as the name indicates - a creative, an activative force through the mental and the physical conditions of the body. Thus there should be, then, the realization that organs and their functionings have become aware, or conscious, of their activity, their function within the system. While as yet this is not a true or full conception, there is the awareness and the awakening of those influences within the system ... (1523-8)

Dr. McGarey states:

"In the first selection, Cayce is saying that the castor oil when applied is active as that which allows the acting together or coordination between the functioning of organs in the system. He indicates elsewhere that in his terminology any acting part of the body is an organ so the nervous system, muscles, etc., would all qualify as organs. The oil assumes this relationship of being the means, perhaps, by which the organs function together only when the activity of the body as a whole is considered, it being directed by higher intelligence. Thus, when one performs an action, oil allows the body to coordinate and act. (Oil, of course, is found within the body, and in a condition of health, the packs would not be needed anyway.) This extract seems to be saying that the oil acts upon the mind forces, or acts to allow the mind forces in the body to become active in producing better coordination between parts of the body and in bringing the spirit into closer communication with the body through these mind forces. Somewhat like putting oil on a wheelbarrow's rusty axle. The wheel will then work in better coordination with the barrow, but it takes the one directing to move it and let the two parts of the wheelbarrow perform better than before their individual functions. The spirit, then, is enhanced in its motivation of the body, through the improved coordination brought about within the parts of that body by the castor oil in its application and action.

The second extract, of course, shows that Cayce believes that consciousness, mind quality, awareness of a particular sort, exists within the very tissues, cells and organs of the body. Thus he sees the castor oil as bringing to the body a closer working together and cooperation between the minds of these tissues or organs, as the body relates to the spirit which motivates it and gives it life.

He does not say in what physical way the oil brings this about, but we can see how such a concept would explain the results which have been attained in practice. Perhaps the autonomic nervous system provides the physical counterpart of the "activity" that Cayce mentions as occurring between the functionings of the organs, and oil, in its vibratory essence becomes the "nature" of that activity, bringing about a better coordination and a resultant bodily function that spells healing to the individual. How can such a concept be simply explained? Cayce involves us with the spirit of life, so we become even more than just body and mind, if he is correct. In any event, this is a credible idea which does give understanding to results obtained, and perhaps gives us a better idea of what sort of conditions might be benefited by such therapy.

What part is played here, then, by the lymph, which has occasioned so much comment thus far? This must be discussed in a summary form, as it relates particularly to the function of the autonomic nervous system, for these are closely related and important one to the other.

Cayce sees the lacteals as that anatomical portion of the body which makes it possible for the body to take values from the food and to prepare these values in such a manner that they can be used to revitalize and bring back to life, so to speak, all the tissues the entire system - of this same body. Moreover, he sees the Peyer's patches as creating a "globular" substance which is carried by the lymphocytes to the contact points between the "sympathetic" and the cerebrospinal nervous systems, which occur in the spinal cord or the sympathetic ganglia which lie anterior to the entire spinal column. This substance is necessary to form a contact between these two systems, and lack of proper contact brings sometimes physical disorders, sometimes mental derangement that varies from very mild to critically serious in its degree. He infers that this lack of contact is a true lack of relationship (in one cell or millions of them) between the physical consciousness and the "soul and spirit forces" - what we may perhaps call the unconscious mind. The implications of this, of course, are rather widespread and drastic, and leave much suggested which cannot be elaborated upon here.

This same area just mentioned - the spinal cord relationship or connection to the sympathetic ganglia - is often the site of difficulty, which Cayce explains as a "lesion" which forms, due to injury or depletion of the system in certain foodstuffs or nutritional needs, or perhaps through stress situations in life. The following selection demonstrates one manner in which the readings see this lesion coming into being, and indicates that it in turn causes trouble to the system."

Cayce states:

In the beginning, then, the cause, or seat of the trouble, we find that there was that in the system that produced a depletion to the physical resistance. During this period there was an injury, or a subluxation, to the 9th and 10th dorsal vertebrae. In the recuperation, in ease, the body formed a lesion to meet the needs of the condition. (943-1)

Dr. McGarey states:

"This philosophy of function in the human body, as becomes gradually apparent in study, would have us understand that these lesions which are formed then become the etiology of other troubles throughout the body, through imperfect transmission of impulses from the higher brain centers to the general areas of the internal workings of the body which are controlled autonomically by the ganglia which are thus affected. We have seen this in numerous selections already quoted. Then a function such as the liver performs is affected, and coordination between the liver and perhaps the kidney as a portion of the elimination of the body becomes a problem. The patient may then develop a frequency or irritation without evidence of infection. Through the disturbance to the liver, the digestion may be affected, and then, in quick order, the assimilation of needed food qualities is limited, the energies of the body suffer, and the nervous system is affected through the lack of substances given to the lymphatic system and subsequent inadequate lymphocytes and again the "globular" substance. So one can see that, in the same manner that "man is not an island", the organs of the body do not stand alone. They are units only in being parts of a larger unit.

Even those many qualities of the world outside of oneself are sensed in such a manner that it becomes effective as an influence on the functioning of the body as a whole. Sounds, colors, tastes, odors, the "feel" of something - all these are shunted through the autonomic nervous system in which manner they become as influences to the organs and tissues of the body as part of their individual consciousness, as these same sensations make their way to consciousness of the whole individual. Even the lesions which occur in the body, as Cayce describes them, become associated with the energies of perception and sensing. In this instance that follows, the lesion is not apparently associated with the spinal cord-ganglion relationship, but rather is one of those created in the abdominal cavity, which may be the type conceivably created by lymphatic disturbance and inadequate lymphatic drainage from a given site. (This does not seem to be quite clear, yet - at least in my studies of the readings.)"

Cayce states:

Question. What happened, a few months ago during the headache, when something seemed to pop in my head, - since which time the attacks haven't seemed to be as severe?
Answer. There is the coordination between the nerve systems, as we have indicated, at the area where the medulla oblongata enters the lower portion or the brain, see? At that period when there was such a severe attack, there was the breaking or a lesion in the abdominal area. This SOUNDED through the sympathetic nerve system, PRODUCING the condition in the head itself. For, as was indicated, it appeared to go THROUGH AND OUT the head. (1857-1)

Dr. McGarey states:

"The emotions, responses within the individual to conditions outside the body in relationship to other people, self's evaluation of self, all bring about within the body a disturbance that often sees certain areas affected according to the emotions experienced. But the balance within the body organs and body systems becomes disturbed, elimination is hindered, intake of food is associated with turmoil, and the beginnings are seen of body sickness through just the mechanisms which have been here only lightly touched upon.

The circulatory system to various parts of the body as it is related to the autonomic is a site of disturbance frequently mentioned. These relationships were not made clear in the study just completed, nor were those which bring together the efficacy of the castor oil packs in pelvic diseases and the sacral parasympathetic supply to these organs.

Much in the way of physiologic function as seen by these readings which Cayce gave for over forty years becomes shifted into the first levels of understandability as serious study is given portions of the readings. The rationale of castor oil pack therapy begins to become apparent. And few, if any, contradictions show up in the rather startling number of words which flowed in such a strange manner from the lips of a dedicated man and the reaches of an unconscious mind.

A rather humorous sidelight on the castor oil pack therapy is the story of a member of the Association for Research and Enlightenment whose wife was developing more and more cervical cysts at the opening of the uterus. He wrote enthusiastically some time later of the wonderful results obtained in clearing up the cysts (as reported by their physician) when they used a circulating file (selections from the readings on a specific condition) and applied the recommendations found there in readings given for various people over the years. The humor lay in the treatment of cervical cysts from the file on cystitis. But it worked - the treatment was castor oil packs as principal therapy.

We begin perhaps, to see that it is not so strange that a castor oil pack can be applied to the abdomen, and in one person a vaginitis is cleared up; in a second case a fecal impaction causing intestinal obstruction is relieved; in a third a threatened abortion is rendered into a normal pregnancy; in a fourth a cholecystitis is cured; and in a fifth, after ten long months, the hair is made to suds and curl once more. Unless physiologic factors were at work that we do not wholly understand, these things could not be.

Cayce, whose work on these readings ceased nearly twenty years ago with his death, would undoubtedly agree that this last extract would speak to these strange results from a strange therapy."

Cayce states:

For, what is the source of all healing for human ills? From whence doth the body receive life, light or immortality? That the body as an active force is the result of spirit and mind, these coordinating and cooperating, enables the entity to bring forth in the experience that which may be used - or the using of the abilities of whatever nature. Each soul has within its power that to use which may make it at one with Creative Forces or God. These are the sources from which life, light, and the activity of the body, mind and soul may manifest in whatever may be the active source or principle in the mind of the individual entity. (3492-1)

Cayce states:

There are then, as given, those influences in the nature of man that may supply that needed. For, man in his nature - physical, mental and spiritual - is a replica, is a part of whole universal reaction in materiality.

Hence there are those elements which if applied in a material way, if there is the activity with same of the spirit and mind, may bring into the experience of each atom of the body force or cell itself the awareness of the Creative Force of God. It may rise only as high as the ideal held by the body-mind.

Hence there is the one way, the source. For in Him is all life, all health, all mind, all knowledge and immortality to the soul-mind itself. (3492-1)

Dr. McGarey states:

"Those who are receptive in their nature will benefit most from the packs. Why is this? Because being receptive is being as the little child. He has faith without even knowing why, and so accepts all things as being the will and the graciousness of God acting in his life. And the peace comes to him, throughout the whole of the earth - his earth.

Healing may really be peace - a peace that comes to rest in the body, that is a reflection of the "peace that passeth understanding". We see it come to the body much as peace is allowed to come to the earth: a nation here and a nation there. When we find real peace in the earth, we may see a state of health having come to all bodies."

It is important to note how many times these words appear in Cayce readings:

Soul – 5347 Documents

Christ – 1424 Documents

Spirit – 2983 Documents

Selfish – 582 Documents

God – 4500 Documents

Interesting work conducted in Japan illustrate how Castor Oil packs affect ones aura. Actual pictures before and after using castor oil, show the nature of this girls aura. According to Mr. Sakaue, a leading authority on auras, this picture shows a very tired person.

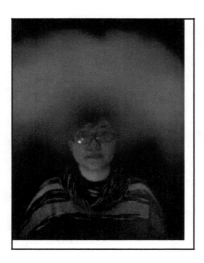

The next picture of the same person in the same place three days later shows, according to Mr. Sakaue, that some kind of purification has taken place in her aura. In other words, he said that three days use of the castor oil seemed to have had a detox affect on her aura.

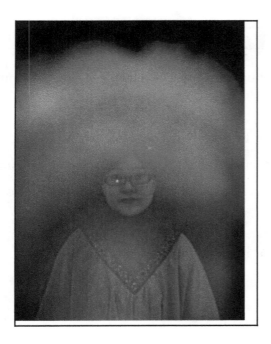

According to the group: We use the castor oil on the liver, and the liver is the organ that tends to store anger energy. When we use a castor oil pack on our liver, it seems to reset our emotional state, and we can regain our true selves.

Chapter Seven: Modern Day Medical Uses – Cancer and Beyond

Castor oil is alive and well. Millions of people world wide know about it and use it. Just Google "castor oil" or "castor oil pack" and see how many vitamin-supplement companies and web sites and blogs pop up. Many medical professionals make use of it today.

A professional who administered Cayce Remedies with great success and acclaim was Dr. Harold Reilly. Dr. Harold Reilly was born on the Lower East Side of New York City in 1895. He served in the United States army with the 102nd engineers. In 1916 he graduated from the National Eclectic Institute. He also earned degrees from Ithaca College and Eastern Reserve University. Dr Reilly also graduated from the American College of Naturopathy and the American School of Chiropractic, and completed two years of study in osteopathy. Considered one of the most renowned physiotherapists in the world, Dr Reilly died in 1987 in Virginia Beach.

What is so fascinating, is the fact that Dr. Reilly knew Edgar Cayce, and received training from him. He used his techniques for 45 years. Dr. Reilly's name came to Edgar Cayce during a trance state and so he began referring patients (over 1000) to him at his world famous clinic called "Reilly Health Institute in New York City's Rockefeller Center. Government and business leaders such as Nelson Rockefeller, David Sarnoff, and George Meany; actors and actresses such as Mickey Rooney, Gloria Swanson, and Leslie Caron; international jet setters such as the Duke and Duchess of Windsor and the Dowager Empress of Egypt; and the famous from all walks of life, from Norman Vincent Peale to Robert Frost; credited Dr. Reilly with helping them to enjoy life to the fullest.

Perhaps his most famous patient, was Bob Hope, the great actor and comedian of years gone by. I often wondered why Bob Hope always looked so young and seemed so healthy, even when he was in his 90's. Dr. Reilly would often travel with Mr. Hope and it was the Cayce methods that helped maintain his good health. This statement that Bob Hope made sums it all up: "Everyone should live the life of Reilly"

Dr. Reilly created the Cayce/Reilly Massage, a particular style of Swedish Massage he developed from information suggested in the Cayce readings. Since the school opened its doors in 1987, more than 1,060 students have graduated from the massage program to share the Cayce healing principles with clients, family, and friends.

Another great medical professional is Dr. John Christopher (1909-1983). He is considered the authority in natural healing with herbs. He created more than 50 herbal formulas and wrote numerous books, all considered classics in the field. His herbal formulas brought about almost miraculous results. He was hailed as America's foremost herbalist in a nationwide survey conducted by Utah Survey

Associates.

Dr. Christopher's mission was to teach people how to cleanse and nourish their bodies so they could heal and prevent disease. Dr. Christopher started The School of Natural Healing in 1953 to teach others natural healing principles. Since that time thousands have benefited from his teachings. Graduates of the School receive a Master Herbalist degree. Master Herbalist's are trusted worldwide for their experience and knowledge.

His world renowned incurables program includes the use of castor oil packs and this program has saved the lives of many. He also used the packs for a number of illnesses with great success.

Its use in modern medicine should be noted:

The United States Food and Drug Administration (FDA) has categorized castor oil as "generally recognized as safe and effective" (GRASE) for over-the-counter use as a laxative with its major site of action the small intestine where it is digested into Ricinoleic acid.

Therapeutically, modern drugs are rarely given in a pure chemical state, so most active ingredients are combined with excipients or additives. Castor oil, or a castor oil derivative such as Kolliphor EL (polyethoxylated castor oil, a nonionic surfactant), is added to many modern drugs, including:

Miconazole, an anti fungal agent;

Paclitaxel, a mitotic inhibitor used in cancer chemotherapy;

Sandimmune (cyclosporine injection, USP), an immunosuppressant drug widely used in connection with organ transplant to reduce the activity of the patient's immune system;

Nelfinavir mesylate, an HIV protease inhibitor;

Saperconazole, a triazole anti fungal agent (contains Emulphor EL-719P, a castor oil derivative);

Tacrolimus, an immunosuppressive drug (contains HCO-60, polyoxyl 60 hydrogenated castor oil);

Xenaderm ointment, a topical treatment for skin ulcers, is a combination of Peru balsam, castor oil, and trypsin;

Aci-Jel (composed of ricinoleic acid from castor oil, with acetic acid and oxyquinoline) is used to maintain the acidity of the vagina.

A topic that often comes up with respect to castor oil pack treatment is its effectiveness with cancer. There are many doctor cases where packs or the oil applied topically cured and helped the disease. Let's look at what Edgar Cayce said about Cancer as reported in the A.R.E. data base (Association For Research and Enlightenment – developed around Edgar Cayce readings)

EDGAR CAYCE'S PERSPECTIVE OF CANCER

Edgar Cayce gave many readings for persons suffering from a wide variety of cancerous conditions. Here are some of the key points to consider with regard to Edgar Cayce's perspective of cancer.

CANCER IS AN ENTITY UNTO ITSELF. In most cases, cancer is a group of cells or tissues which separates ("segregates") itself and forms its own entity within the larger system of the body. In a sense, cancer has its own separate identity like a parasite which infests a host organism.

CANCER REPRESENTS A FAILURE OF NATURAL PROCESSES. Edgar Cayce observed that the same processes which result in cancer are present in the body all the time. Cancer usually results from the failure of natural processes such as coagulation and elimination of wastes.

CANCER DRAWS FROM THE VITALITY OF THE BODY. Cancer uses the body's life-force energy to survive. Like any parasite, cancer is a drain upon the resources of the host organism.

CANCER HAS MANY CAUSES. There are many etiological (causative) factors associated with cancer. Heredity, environmental toxicity, poor eliminations, injury, lack of vitality, and depleted immune system were the most often cited factors linked to cancer. Specifically, chronic irritation or bruising were often said to be triggering factors producing tumors which could become malignant.

THERE ARE MANY FORMS OF CANCER. Edgar Cayce recognized the various kinds of cancer. On two occasions he stated that there are nineteen forms of cancer.

CANCER CAN OFTEN BE PREVENTED. According to Edgar Cayce, keeping a healthy diet and good eliminations can help prevent cancer. Specific therapies such as iodex and ash ointment and plantain salve were recommended by Cayce to prevent lumps and tumors from becoming malignant. Gentle osteopathic treatment was also often prescribed to set up "drainages" and improve eliminations thus decreasing the chances for cancer.

EARLY TREATMENT RESULTS IN BETTER PROGNOSIS. In agreement with modern medicine's view of cancer treatment, Edgar Cayce noted that early intervention produces better therapeutic results.

CANCER INVOLVES MENTAL AND SPIRITUAL ASPECTS. Edgar Cayce's holistic approach to health and healing is notable in the readings he gave for person's suffering from cancer. The mental and spiritual aspects of prevention and treatment were strongly emphasized. Cayce also stated that excessive worry and negative attitudes can make a person with a genetic predisposition for cancer more vulnerable to developing the illness.

CANCER IS SOMETIMES A KARMIC PATTERN. Consistent with the perennial philosophy which acknowledges the continuity of consciousness, Edgar Cayce observed that in some cases cancer can result from past life experiences.

THE TREATMENT OF CANCER INVOLVES MANY MODALITIES. Edgar Cayce recommended a wide variety of therapeutic modalities for the treatment of cancer. Treatments directed at decreasing toxicity and increasing vitality were emphasized. On the whole, natural therapies that worked with the body to heal itself were given priority.

EDGAR CAYCE SOMETIMES RECOMMENDED SURGERY AND RADIATION. In certain cases where the cancer was progressive and extreme, surgery and/or radiation therapy were recommended. Modern chemotherapy techniques were not available during Edgar Cayce's era.

SOME CASES OF CANCER WERE REGARDED AS INCURABLE. Although Edgar Cayce was generally optimistic with regard to the body's innate ability to heal itself from almost any illness, in some cases of cancer the disease was too advanced to expect a physical cure. In such instances, Cayce would recommend therapies to decrease the pain and suffering while emphasizing the mental/spiritual (soul) aspects of healing.

There are many instances of cancer cures using Cayce suggestions, including castor oil packs and castor oil applied to spots on the body. The one that follows was told to Dr. McGarey during an A.R.E. Conference:

"My husband and I took part in the Temple Beautiful Program in 1992 due to Tom's having prostate cancer. His surgeon stated that he wanted to operate again; otherwise Tom had only four months to live.

After arriving at the A.R.E. Clinic and entering the Temple Beautiful Program, Tom kept up with the meditation, castor oil packs, diet program and exercises.

One day after I returned home, Tom told me that he did not have cancer any longer. He removed the castor oil pack and displayed the flannel that looked like a rag with green, black and brown spots all over the surface. Every toxin had been removed out of his body onto the castor oil flannel.

He went on to live another four years with no cancer symptoms. A couple of months before he died, he realized he had not urinated in twenty-four hours. As you know when the bladder is full, it lets you feel the discomfort. Tom did not have a pressure or pain and after CAT scans were diagnosed, they revealed that his kidney had stopped functioning. The scans also showed no cancer in his mid-section of the body. What had caused his death were the adhesions caused by the radiation treatments."

Another case reported by Dr. McGarey:

"A researcher tells the story of a thirty-three-year-old women who developed terminal cancer two years ago after a radical mastectomy. Her therapy had included surgery, radiation, cobalt and belatron treatments, and chemotherapy involving five FU. Her condition became serious: she developed peptic ulcers, elimination problems, and abdominal distention. Becoming disoriented and out of touch with reality, she was hospitalized. She now started on castor oil packs over the entire abdomen. Her urinary tract started working again, and the distention gradually subsided while still impacted. On the fourth day, she finally started having bowel activity. On the fifth day, she had her first regular bowel movement in weeks. Her hallucinations cleared up, her vision improved considerably, and she was able to go home.

Castor oil packs did not clear up the malignancy we call cancer, but it did aid the sensorium in this women and brought about significant improvement of the elimination and the total experience of her treatments."

This case was reported in the Heritage Publication, the year was 2000 (Article: Edgar Cayce Products – Thirty Years of Research):

"I have a friend named Jake, who has also found the amazing curative powers of the oil when used externally. He was sitting home one night when his mother phoned from Green Bay, Wisconsin. She informed him that he had to come home as soon as possible, as his father was dying, Jake was stunned because the last he had heard his father, seventy-one, was in fine health. His father has to go for his automobile insurance, and they would not insure him unless he had a physical. After examining him, the doctors discovered that he had high blood pressure. It came as quite a shock to Jake's father since he felt particularly well. Therefore, the doctors put him on those lethal blood pressure pills and in nine months, he developed cancer, emphysema and diabetes. Jake arrived home in tow days, and arrived at the hospital to see his father lying in bed, down from 145 pounds to 98 pounds. Unable to recognize his son, or anything else for that matter, it would be only a matter of hours before he died. Jake phoned me in Los Angeles and said to look in the Black Book and see what Cayce had to say about the aforementioned diseases. I said that I did not see anything about them. He hung up the phone, angry, then went running to the drug store where he bought a bottle of castor oil. He then applied the oil over his father's body from his neck to his thighs. He did not even use a heating pad or hot compresses, as Cayce had recommended , and as we had both used in the past. The following morning, his father opened his eyes and exclaimed, "Jake, when did you get home?" A couple of hours later he was sitting up in bed. The nurse came, but she was not surprised. This often happens, she said with terminal patients. Jake's father did not die. Instead he started going to the bathroom by himself for the first time in six weeks. By the end of the week, he was eating at the dining room table and talking of spending the winter in Florida. Jake left soon after he realized his father was improving and that was only after a single castor oil application. I have discovered that the more serious the condition, the faster castor oil will work."

Another story based upon a personal interview recorded by the A.R.E.:

I know of an individual who was diagnosed with two forms of cancer, a lymphoma and melanoma. He had a heart attack the year before and was HIV positive. When he came in, he asked, "Can you help me?" and I thought, "What don't you have?" I could see that he was really quite frightened. After listening to this man's story, he was such a laid-back person; it shocked me that he would have had a heart attack. He was not an uptight appearing nor stressed individual. It was suggested that he do the castor oil packs, leaving them on all night, just sleeping with the pack.

He had some funny stories to tell about his experience using the castor oil packs. He would wake up in the middle of the night and discover his pack had slipped out of place pushing up around his neck, and in that position, it became quite disorienting.

Nevertheless, he finally figured out how to keep it in place. He did the castor oil pack, changed his diet towards alkalizing his system and used one of Cayce's green rays with carbon ash, as well as meditated daily. Definitely castor oil every night, seven days a week, he wore the pack.

At the end of the month, he was supposed to go back for another examination, as the doctors were to set him up with a protocol of all kinds of stuff. At the finalization of the tests, they could not find any Melanoma. They had done biopsies so it was not their guessing-they had taken samples and diagnosed him. They only found one lymph node in his side that was suspicious so they took that out. However, the doctor at the time asked, "Are you a religious man?" He said "No, why do you ask?" and the doctor said, "Well, God loves you. Anyone of two or three things that you had could have gotten you". In addition, his immune system was back up in high normal so I know the castor oil had something to do with that because we had worked with other AIDS patients and the ones that had used it regularly, their immune system did return."

Some more cases Dr. McGarey reports about:

Castor oil has been used widely in instances of skin cancer. With regard to the skin ... a man about 68 years old had a mean-looking lesion on his ear which was probably an early squamous cell carcinoma; biopsy was not done. This lesion had been present for years. The patient has had basal cell carcinoma removed from the area of the left ear somewhat near this particular lesion. At any rate, after two weeks of the castor oil and camphorated oil, the lesion disappeared and has not recurred. The treatment was started in December of 1969.

Another patient, a woman of 61, had a lesion inside her ear in the external auditory meatus, which was rough and scaly, and she used the castor oil-camphorated oil. The lesion disappeared and has maintained its absence after about three weeks of treatment. No recurrence since April 22. This lesion had been bleeding a bit, and this I think makes the result with the oil combination even more dramatic.

A 58-year-old Oklahoma woman tells the story of how her skin cancers bothered her constantly for more than 15 years, until she started applying one of the Cayce remedies for such problems. Her face was the site of the trouble. She stayed out of the sun or wore a wide-brimmed hat to shade the sun from her skin. But when she discovered what to do, things began to change. Here is her story:

"There was a tiny bump on my forehead which never healed. It formed a scab, it came off, bled a little, formed another scab, ad infinitum. I finally mixed 2 teaspoons full of castor oil with 1 teaspoonful of baking soda and placed some of this on the irritated place, covering it with a Band-Aid. In three days, the irritation disappeared from sight but not from touch. I could still feel it. At the end of two more days treating it like this, it was gone and has not recurred."

Here is an example of Cayce's approach to breast cancer. Note the reference to "prenatal" (hereditary) factors which is documented by a family history of cancer.

Cayce: Yes, we have the body here. This we have had before. Conditions are not so well with the body as when we last had same here. Those conditions as are prenatal in their effect, through the activity of forces made manifest in a physical body, are beginning to become in the manner of producing within the system an element as of its OWN resuscitation, living upon the life OF the body-physical. That's a very good description of cancer, isn't it? for it IS malignant in its nature, and has already attacked the mammary glands, and is going to be rather fast in its operation unless there are means taken as to check same. (2457-4)

This woman was 38 years old when this reading was given. She followed the treatment recommended in her readings and was cured of her cancer. She lived for another 36 years, dying in in her sleep at the age of 74.

Chapter Eight
The A.R.E. - The Association for Research and Enlightenment

The Association for Research and Enlightenment was founded by Edgar Cayce in 1931. The official address is as follows: 215 67th Street, Virginia Beach, VA 23451 (Toll free: 800-333-4499; 757-428-3588). Their web link is: **www.edgarcayce.org**

Their mission is to explore holistic health, spirituality, intuition, dreams, psychic development, reincarnation and ancient mysteries. These are subjects that Edgar Cayce addressed in his more than 14,000 documented readings. Their mission statement is worth noting and is quite beautiful:

> The Mission of the A.R.E. is to help people transform their lives for the better, through research, education, and application of core concepts found in the Edgar Cayce readings and kindred materials that seek to manifest the love of God and all people and promote the purposefulness of life, the oneness of God, the spiritual nature of humankind, and the connection of body, mind, and spirit.

Overseeing a worldwide effort, the association has regional headquarters in Houston, regional representatives throughout the U.S., and Edgar Cayce Centers in 37 countries. More than 70 countries have A.R.E. members. It oversees: A.R.E. conferences, international tours, camps for children and adults, regional activities, and study groups that allow like-minded people to gather for educational and fellowship opportunities worldwide.

A.R.E. offers membership benefits and services that include a quarterly body-mind-spirit member magazine, Venture Inward; a member newsletter covering the topics of ancient mysteries, personal spirituality, and holistic health. Member fees are minimal, as low as $20 per year for students and a little more for adults. The value of this is priceless, since the money is going to a worthy non profit cause and with the membership one can access Cayce's readings on line with a powerful search tool, which makes it easy to find information on any topic in a matter of seconds.

A.R.E.'s publishing arm, A.R.E. Press, began publishing books in 1931, and has since branched out into DVDs, CDs, ebooks, and digital media. In 2009, the organization launched a second imprint, 4th Dimension Press, in order to offer additional like-minded materials. Individuals can purchase A.R.E. Press/4th Dimension Press products in nearly any bookstore or online at ARECatalog.com. Edgar Cayce's A.R.E. also maintains an affiliation with Atlantic University, which offers continuing education classes and a master's degree program in Transpersonal Studies; the Cayce/Reilly® School of Massotherapy, a leader in holistic education, wellness, and healthcare; and maintains an on site Health

Center & Spa at its Virginia Beach headquarters, where many of the health readings remedies are offered along with massage therapy.

The A.R.E. Library - Virginia Beach, Va.

The Edgar Cayce A.R.E. Library stands as a living memorial to the life and work of Edgar Cayce, whose more than 14,000 psychic readings form the core of the collection. In addition to the Cayce readings, the Library houses one of the largest collections in the world - 65,000 volumes - specializing in the fields of metaphysics, parapsychology, comparative religious studies, holistic health, ancient civilizations, and foreign language editions of Edgar Cayce books.

Edgar Cayces vision of the library states:

To provide library service, enhance spiritual community, strengthen connectedness within the Association, foster personal growth, encourage "the love of God and man," and promote the oneness of all life in the experience of those who seek greater consciousness. "All knowledge is to be used in the manner that will give help and assistance to others, and the desire is that the laws of the Creator be manifested in the physical world." - Edgar Cayce

Cayce also states:

"The purpose, then, of the Association: The institution [is to be] built around that of a place where the records of that accomplished through these sources are kept, and others of similar nature, or of the various philosophies that may be found that will coordinate-and combined in that oneness of purpose to bring the better understanding of the purpose in life, and thus enable man to realize the closer association with the divine. In the lecture room and the library-members, then, having access to such, gain better in the understanding of such, and the library may be made circulating, or a repository-as it will become-to all those who seek to see their theory disseminated. Hence this would become as the clearing house of such."
(Edgar Cayce reading #254-37)

The A.R.E. is involved in world wide research, some of which was mentioned on national TV with respect to Edgar Cayce's pronouncements regarding the location of Atlantis. Ongoing site investigation for Atlantis, based upon Cayce's work, will no doubt yield spectacular results over time.

Chapter Nine: Where To Buy and How To Use The Oil

Before getting into the specifics of what product to buy, where to find it, and how to use it, a question should be addressed: "Under what circumstances do I use it and when should it not be used?"

As a general rule of thumb it can be used for any health problem – internal or external, at any time. It should not be used if fever is present and if you are pregnant unless so advised by your doctor. Many women have used it to save their pregnancy and to help conceive. But it can have the opposite effect when taken internally, and actually help induce labor. It can latch on to the walls of the small intestine and cause contractions. As with any health issue, please consult your health care provider before using castor oil externally or internally.

Edgar Cayce suggested it be used externally in most of his readings, but its internal use is of value. Remember that castor oil has been sold and used over the counter as a laxative for many centuries. Dr. McGarey relates a wonderful story of how its internal use had remarkable health benefits normally not associated with a laxative:

"Early in my use of castor oil packs in the practice of medicine, I had an interesting experience which taught me something about the real nature of the cells that go to make up this body of ours. I had been treating a woman for anemia. She had a hemoglobin of 9.3 grams (significantly below the norm). I had given her a product called Feosol, which supplies extra iron and was indicated for the anemia.

She returned six weeks later and I checked her hemoglobin again. It was still 9.3 grams. This time, however, she had a skin rash. It was not severe, but bothersome. Iron taken by mouth frequently causes a skin rash, and this was what appeared to be happening. I had read in the literature about a dermatologist who had given his patients castor oil by mouth which had cleared up the skin. So I suggested to this woman that she stop the iron and take an ounce of castor oil that night, repeat it in four days, and then let me see her again She didn't really hear me about the time factor, so she showed up in another six weeks. She had felt so good that she kept on taking the castor oil every four days. I checked her skin. It was clear, of course. Her hemoglobin was next. Without the iron by mouth and with no other medication directed toward the anemia, her hemoglobin had risen to 13.4 and was normal. What happened? Apparently the oil cleansed the cells that lined the upper intestinal tract where iron is absorbed from the food normally, and the body overcame its problem of iron deficiency. Cleansing, not iron tablets, healed the body."

One can find castor oil in almost any store – supermarket, drug store, department store, health food store. Unfortunately you should only buy the oil if it is organic (cold pressed) and as such, will be hexane free. Hexane is a chemical used to extract oil from its seed.

When locating castor oil the manufacture date is important to make note of, but is not a big factor when purchasing the oil. It is almost impossible to buy castor oil that is outdated, since quality product sells so fast that it will never sit on the shelf for more than one month at most. Castor oil has a long shelf life, as long as it smells good and looks clear it usually is okay to use. It can last 2-3 years and should be kept in a cold dark place – the refrigerator allows it to last longer.

Because this is a health related item always use fresh oil. If your oil has been sitting around for months buy some fresher product. It is very inexpensive.

The A.R.E. has an official source that it refers people to: www.baar.com Baar sells a wide variety of health products, including all the Edgar Cayce remedies. The castor oil they sell is cold pressed and hexane free.

Another company that sells the oil is The Heritage Store: www.heritagestore.com They carry all the Cayce products as well.

Both Baar and The Heritage Store sell their products on Amazon.com

A number of third party vendors have good quality product at low prices, often 50 % less than companies like Baar and Heritage. Again, make sure it is cold pressed and hexane free.

When using the oil as a pack it needs to be applied to a material then placed on the skin. Cayce recommended wool or cotton flannel. It can be purchased along with the oil from any of the sources listed above. It should be pure in form – non bleached, so pay the extra for quality. A larger size piece should be purchased, say 12 inches by 28 inches, because it needs to be folded into at least 3 thicknesses, according to Cayce. The final size should be about 12 inches square, bigger person bigger size, smaller person smaller size.

It is best to purchase a 32 oz size (one quart) of castor oil, enough for at least one-two people for 4-6 weeks of treatment.

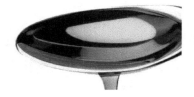

TYPICAL PLACEMENT OF CASTOR OIL PACK

Although castor oil packs can be used on almost any area of the body, the most common placement is over the right side of the abdomen from the liver to the caecum. The liver is on the right side where the bottom of the rib cage is – just feel your ribs to see.

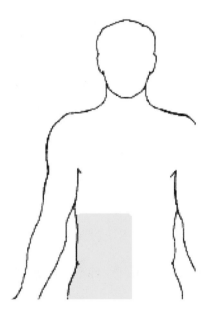

The A.R.E. has prepared a you tube video that demonstrates the use of the castor oil pack. This link and all references in this book will be provided in the supplemental material.

What the video demonstrates is to place the castor oil pack (oil soaked flannel or cotton cloth) over the liver-stomach area on the right side and cover with plastic, then heat using a heating pad (as hot as you can stand), then a towel to hold it all in place. Lie down and relax while doing it. Remember, as the video states, the oil soaked flannel must be saturated with oil but not dripping.

The general rule of thumb is to use the packs for three nights in a row at the same time each night for 1 – 1 ½ hours at a time. Wait four days then do it again. So basically you are doing it each week at the same time. From 4-6 weeks, is the usual duration. After each treatment a small amount of olive oil is recommended – start with ½ teaspoon then work up to maybe a tablespoon. Some recommend waiting until after the third treatment before taking the olive oil. The olive oil is very important as it helps stimulate the liver to dump toxins out of the system. Remember that Edgar Cayce's suggestions for use varied somewhat for each person. So hard and fast rules cannot be applied here. Follow your instincts. If for example, after one hour, you become uncomfortable, stop. Some use the packs for more than three days in a row.

After using a castor oil pack store the flannel in a plastic bag in the refrigerator. It can be used over and over again, as long as it appears clean and smells okay. If it appears discolored in any way, get rid of it. It can last for months. Remember the golden rule that applies to food and it applies here as well: "When in doubt, through it out!"

The castor oil pack can be applied to any part of the body, so if a problem area appears do not hesitate to place a pack over it. Castor oil can be applied topically by itself or mixed with baking soda to form a paste. Just pour some oil into a cup and add some baking soda until it mixes into a thick paste (50-50 mix). It is easy to apply the oil this way. Dr. McGarey suggests these types of applications:

- Five drops of castor oil orally each morning to control allergies.
- Puncture wounds, cuts and bruises heal rapidly when rubbed with castor oil.
- Prevention of pregnancy stretch marks when abdomen is rubbed with castor oil during the last two months of pregnancy.
- Rapid healing of a sprained ankle wrapped overnight in castor oil.
- Marked reduction in tinnitus and hearing loss by applying castor oil drops in the ears.
- Rapid healing of hepatitis using daily castor oil packs.
- Clearing of cataracts with one drop of castor oil in each eye at bedtime.
- Healing of a pilonidal cyst after castor oil packs.
- Clearing of brown skin aging spots with castor oil plus baking soda.
- Relief of severe eye allergies by rubbing eyelids with castor oil at bedtime.
- Relief of low back pain with one week of castor oil packs.
- Relief of chronic diarrhea with abdominal castor oil packs.
- Clearing of vocal cord nodes & hoarseness with castor oil packs daily on the neck for 3 months.
- Complete clearing of tinnitus with 6-8 drops of castor oil orally each day for four weeks.
- Clearing of hyperactivity with abdominal castor oil packs.
- Removal of a wart after four weeks of application of castor oil.
- Resolution of a calcium deposit from the sole of the foot with daily castor oil massage.
- Clearing of skin cancer with castor oil plus baking soda.
- Clearing of snoring after two weeks of abdominal castor oil packs.
- Rapid clearing of a bee sting by application of castor oil.
- Increased hair growth with daily scalp massage with castor oil twenty minutes before shampooing.
- Clearing of nail fungus after four months of castor oil packs on the nail.

After using the oil make sure you rub it off using 2 teaspoons of baking soda in 2 quarts of warm water. Some like to shower afterwards and use soap, then the baking soda-water mix to clean the area. The area must be cleaned because castor oil when left on too long produces an acid affect on the body. This rule applies to castor oil packs – leaving it on skin problems for long periods is okay.

This chart mentions other ways to use castor oil:

CONDITION/SYMPTOM	CASTOR OIL REMEDY
Adhesions	Apply castor oil packs.
Age Spots (Brown Skin)	Rub castor oil and baking soda (half-half mixture) into age spot.
Allergies	Five (5) drops of castor oil orally (swallow) each morning will control allergies.
Arthritis	Rub castor oil into the affected area.
Back Pain	Apply castor oil packs for one week.
Bee Sting	Apply castor oil to the sting site.
Blood Clot	Apply castor oil packs.
Cataracts	Place one drop of castor oil in each eye at bedtime (use USP castor oil).
Cuts/Bruises/Wounds	Heal rapidly when rubbed with castor oil.
Diarrhoea	Relieve chronic diarrhoea with abdominal castor oil packs.
Eye Allergies	Rub eyelids with castor oil at bedtime.
Gall Bladder Disease	Using castor oil packs relieves symptoms.
Hair Loss	Daily scalp massage with castor oil – 20 minutes before shampooing hair.
Hearing Loss	Apply castor oil drops in the ears.
Hepatitis	Use daily castor oil packs on the stomach.
Hyperactivity	Use castor oil packs.
Knee Swelling	Wrap the knee in a castor oil cloth overnight.
Menstrual Pain	Use castor oil packs for 6 weeks, or until pain subsides.
Mole	Mix castor oil and baking soda (half-half mixture). Apply to mole until it shrinks and disappears. Castor oil can also remove a mole when used by itself.
Nail Fungus	Place castor oil packs on the nail for a period of around 4 months.
Pregnancy Stretch Marks	Rub abdomen with castor oil during the last two months of pregnancy.
Scleroderma	Apply castor oil packs (this has led to a total cure in one patient).
Skin Cancer	Apply castor oil and baking soda (half-half mixture).
Skin Tag	Mix castor oil and baking soda (half-half mixture). Apply to skin tag until it shrinks and disappears (usually 4-6 weeks).
Snoring	Apply abdominal castor oil packs for around 2 weeks.
Sprained Ankle	Rub with castor oil, or use castor oil packs.
Tinnitus	Swallow 6-8 drops of castor oil each day for 4 weeks.
Varicose Veins	Massage castor oil into irritated varicose veins, and they virtually disappear.
Viral Infections And Flu	Soak in the bathtub for 30 minutes, using 1 cup castor oil in comfortably hot water. Or apply castor oil over the entire body after a shower, then put on an old sweat-suit, tracksuit or long pyjamas (top and bottom) and leave on overnight.
Warts	Apply castor oil for a period of around 4 weeks.

Chapter Ten: Conclusion

Can a health product that has had so many positive results for so many centuries be an anomaly? It is a freak of nature? Or perhaps, it is a product that God gifted to humanity and its vibratory nature is in sync with a higher force and Jesus knew this, and made use of it, and in so doing helped bless it. What does man need from his creator that he hasn't already received? We have life, understanding, mental capacity, and a natural and spiritual environment that provides the nourishment our bodies need to stay healthy and be in tune with the needs of the age in which we live. And when we get a little out of balance, castor oil can help provide the grease, to get the wheel moving freely again.

No one knows for sure how the human body works, what it really needs, or just why we are here on this earth. Religion teaches that we have higher purpose and that our soul is the animating force behind our body and when we feed the body-soul with the right foods, thoughts, and actions, a perfect balance is achieved.

Edgar Cayce really deserves the credit here. I am pretty sure that without his pronouncements on the use of castor oil we would not be having this interchange. And what did he really stand for and what did he really want each of us to achieve, and is it any different from what Jesus wanted and all of God's messengers wanted?

I would like to end with a number of Edgar Cayce quotations and readings (they provide food for thought, or should I say, nourishment for the soul) and finally with a commentary on the concept of "Oneness" that was so important to Edgar Cayce, and in my humble opinion should be the focus of our attention as we go forward as individuals, and as nations seeking health and harmony.

Edgar Cayce Quotations and Answers To Questions:

For all healing-mental and material-is attuning each atom of the body, each reflex of the brain to an awareness of the Divine which lies within each cell

Know that all healing forces are within, not without! The applications from without are merely to create within a coordinating mental and spiritual force.

Remember, the body does gradually renew itself constantly. Do not look upon the conditions which have existed as not being able to be eradicated from the system. Hold to that KNOWLEDGE-and don't think of it as just therapy-that the body CAN, the body DOES, renew itself!

Well that each member of the Board first, each member of the office, each member of the staff, each member of the Association - Associate, Active, Living Sponsor or what - be asked to give at least once each day a silent prayer that the work, the power, the might which may be that guiding force, may bring health, hope, a better understanding of the purpose of life. Ask that the life of Edgar Cayce be spared to serve, to be the greater channel, that the love of God in Christ-Jesus be manifested in the earth; not to the glory or honor of any individual but to the glory and honor of God.

Extracts from reading: 99-8

(Question) How can I use my abilities at the present time to best serve humanity?

(Answer) By filling to the best possible purpose AND ability that place, that niche the body, mind AND soul occupies; being the BEST husband, the best neighbor, the BEST friend to each and every individual the body meets; for would one fail in meeting those obligations that one takes, they become worse THAN the infidel; and as was said, "He that would cause the least of these my little ones to offend, BETTER were it that a millstone be hanged about his neck and he cast in the depths of the sea" - but he that doeth the will of the Father, he that is willing to become as naught that they may SERVE the better in WHATEVER capacity as a merchant, be the best merchant; as a neighbor, the BEST neighbor; as a friend, the BEST friend.

(Question) Give any advice or counsel that will help me to carry out the purpose for which I came into the earth?

(Answer) Little by little does ONE come to the understanding of the PURPOSE for which they came into the earth. Purpose is of the MAKINGS of the individual, PLUS that GIVEN in the beginning, and as souls seek the Father, in that companionship that one may have through communion with Him - and communion with Him means DOING; not shutting self away from thine brother, from thine neighbor, even from thine self - rather APPLYING self to the duties material, mental AND spiritual, as IS known. One would say that "I would do - my body will not allow me to do." This was oft said of old by those who gave themselves in no uncertain manner, but there remains that advocate with the Father, through DOING - and be not WEARY IN well-doing; rather let it be said of thee as of David of old, "Though He slay me, yet will I serve Him the better; though He forsake me, yet will I draw the closer." As one does THOSE things to his neighbor, to his wife, to his friend, to his foe, may the knowledge, the understanding, the BLESSING of life flow in.

Extracts from reading: 262-129

(Question) Please give the affirmation for the next lesson.

(Answer) The next lesson as we find that would be well here, following this, would be: GOD - LOVE - MAN. The affirmation for such would be: LET THAT LIGHT BE WITHIN ME IN SUCH MEASURES THAT I, AS A CHILD OF GOD, MAY REALIZE HIS LOVE FOR MAN. MAY I LIVE THAT, THEN, IN MY LIFE DAY BY DAY.

(Question) Would you give any basic thoughts for this lesson?

(Answer) In this period of man's experience in the earth there is the greater need that he, man, consider the purposes (and the needs) of God in his daily life. There is the need for such thought, such meditation on this universal consciousness, this field, to be manifested by man's love, man's activity towards his fellow man. For, the basic truth that must be presented throughout the study of this subject, is:

"Inasmuch as ye do it unto the least of thy brethren, ye do it unto thy Maker." Man's ability, man's consciousness, man's thought - then - must be directed more and more, - by those in authority, those in power, those as leaders, those as teachers, those as fathers and mothers, those as associates one with another, - to those principles, GOD - LOVE - MAN.

We are through for the present.

Chapter Eleven: The Edgar Cayce Readings On Oneness

The first lesson for six months should be One-One-One- One; Oneness of God, oneness of man's relation, oneness of force, oneness of time, oneness of purpose, Oneness in every effort-Oneness-Oneness!

Edgar Cayce Reading 900-429

What did Cayce mean by oneness? Kevin J Todeschi, as quoted on the EdgarCayce.org web site and adapted from: "Twelve Lessons in Personal Spirituality", gives a brilliant explanation on this subject and it is quoted, in part, here:

"One of the great ironies of human nature is the fact that the very structure intended to enrich our relationship with God is the one thing which divides us most as a human family. For countless eons, more wars have been fought on religious principles than for any other reason. Even to this day, wars, bloodshed, political battles, and countless examples of our inhumanity to one another are commonplace as one group tries to instill (or enforce) its belief systems, its politics, or the supremacy of its God onto the lives of others.

These conflicts are not simply between various religions but are also within each denomination. There are sects within Christianity, Buddhism, Judaism, Hinduism, Islam-within every religion!-many convinced that they are just a little more right than anyone else. Even various churches, temples, and synagogues have found differences with other members of their own sect who have somehow fallen away from the "original" or the "true" faith.

In addition to separating people from one another, these conflicts have also caused individuals to become disillusioned with religion - some even becoming convinced that religion is a waste of time. Too often, the result has been that people have given up their faith in God because of their disappointment in humankind.

Interestingly enough, the Edgar Cayce material states that part of the problem is due to our ignorance of our oneness with one another.

WHERE IS thine OWN will? One with HIS, or to the glorifying of thine own desires -- thine own selfish interests? Edgar Cayce Reading 900-429

Cayce's information presents a hopeful and inspiring approach to spirituality and religion that inextricably weaves all of humanity together. Rather than focusing upon the form of specific religions or dogmas, the readings instead focus upon the importance of every single soul attempting to manifest an awareness of the living Spirit in the earth.

From Cayce's perspective, our goal is not to simply wait for heaven or to escape the earth; instead, we are challenged to bring an awareness of the Creator into our lives and into our surroundings wherever we may be, right now.

> "what is the difference? ...Truth...is of the One source. Are there not trees of oak, of ash, of pine? There are the needs of these for meeting this or that experience...Then, all will fill their place. Find not fault with any, but rather show forth as to just how good a pine, or ash, or oak, or vine thou art!"
> Edgar Cayce Reading 254-87

There is a common bond we all share as a collective humanity: There is but one God, and we are all God's children. In order to reawaken that sense of connectedness we share with one another, the readings state that the start of any spiritual journey should begin with the knowledge that the Lord God is One. Regardless of the name we call God or the religion on earth that we feel drawn to, there is but one Creator, one Source, one Law. In fact, perhaps more than anything else, this concept of "oneness" is the underlying philosophy of the Edgar Cayce readings.

This notion of oneness in a world so filled with variety may, at first, seem a difficult concept to comprehend. After all, we are surrounded by a myriad of plants, trees, animals, experiences, and people. Rather than attempting to make all things the same, however, oneness suggests instead that we have the opportunity to view this rich diversity as an example of the multiple ways in which the One Spirit tries to find expression in our lives. Since there is only one God-the source of all that exists-ultimately, the universe must be composed of only one Force.

Oneness as a force implies that all things are interrelated. Every one of us has a connection to one another, the earth, the universe, and to God. This one force is a force for good which is attempting to bring the spirituality of the Creator into the earth. Unfortunately, because of our limited awareness of the power of free will, individuals are able to direct that force into selfish purposes and desires, creating "evil" in the process.

In terms of spirituality, the concept of oneness suggests that God is not limited to expressing through one religion alone. Instead, the Creator manifests in individuals' lives because of their faith and because of their relationship to the spiritual Source, not because of their specific religion. From Cayce's perspective, religion is the form in which individuals attempt to understand the manifestation of this Spirit. God can (and does!) work through every soul in the earth.

The good news is that, in spite of how things may appear in the world today, the readings assert that all of Creation will eventually be brought into an awareness of this oneness and of the Law of Love which it implies. One of our challenges as individuals is to make the world a better place because we have lived in it. Perhaps the best approach to this consciousness is reflected in the Bible when it states that we must love God with all our heart, mind, and soul, and our neighbor as ourselves.

As a means of discovering the oneness of Spirit, the readings encourage comparative religious study. Through such a discipline, each of us might see beyond surface differences and, instead, find the commonalities we share with one another:

...coordinate the teachings, the philosophies of the east, and the west, the oriental and the occidental, the new truths and the old... Correlate not the differences, but where all religions meet- there is one God! "Know, O Israel, the Lord God is one!"
Edgar Cayce Reading 991-1

...consider a field of corn. In the grain of corn there is life. Man plants it in the soil, works it, and then he reaps the harvest. Not every man selects the same kind of corn. Not every man plows it alike. Not every man sows it alike. Not every man reaps it alike. Yet, in each case it brings forth the very best that there is. It is the God or the life within each grain that the man is seeking. It sustains his body, and also produces enough seed to raise more. That's religion. That's the denominations.
Edgar Cayce Reading 991-1

Since the purpose of life is to bring the spirituality of the Creator into the earth, attunement and application are at the heart of spiritual growth. Attunement is the process of reawakening to an awareness of our spiritual nature and our true relationship with God. As mentioned previously, the most frequently recommended tools for achieving this attunement are the regular practice of prayer and meditation. Both prayer and meditation are invaluable at reestablishing a conscious awareness of our spiritual source while inviting God's will to work through us as a "channel of His blessings" in service to others.

Repeatedly, a core concept from the Edgar Cayce material has been stated: Spirit is the life, mind is the builder, and the physical is the result. In terms of oneness, essentially what this means is that the one force, Spirit, constantly flows through us. However, it is acted upon by the properties of the mind and then channeled into our lives in accordance with our free will. Regardless of whether or not an individual even believes in God, everything about that person is given life through the properties of the one activating Spirit. What he or she does with that Spirit is a matter of choice, and "crimes or miracles" may be the result.

This ability of personal creation, whether through thought, experience or activity, caused the readings to identify the human soul as a cocreator with God. Because of this gift of cocreation, Cayce continually advised individuals that one of the most important things they could do was to establish an appropriate spiritual motivation (or ideal) for their lives, thereby directing personal choice into positive directions. From Cayce's perspective, too often, we are out of touch with the intentionality (the why) behind our everyday actions. By consciously establishing a spiritual motivation, such as service, compassion, love, or Jesus, as our pattern and then trying to make that motivation a greater part of our lives, real personal transformation and soul development can result.

The soul, then, must return-will return-to its Maker. It is a portion of the Creative Force, which is energized into activity even in materiality, in the flesh...Then, just being kind, just being patient, just showing love for thy fellow man; that is the manner in which an individual works at becoming aware of the consciousness or the Christ Spirit. Edgar Cayce Reading 272-9

Each soul in entering the material experience does so for those purposes of advancement towards that awareness of being fully conscious of the oneness with the Creative Forces. Edgar Cayce Reading 2632-1

Oneness as a force suggests that each of us is connected in ways that we might never before have imagined. Our challenge is to bring that wholeness to consciousness, an "awareness within each soul, imprinted in pattern on the mind and waiting to be awakened by the will, of the soul's oneness with God." (5749-14) Regardless of an individual's religion or personal beliefs, this Christ pattern exists in potential upon the very fiber of his or her being. It is that part which is in perfect accord with the Creator and is simply waiting to find manifestation in one's life."

The founder of the Baha'i Faith, Baha'u'llah, said it best, when speaking about the oneness of mankind:

"Ye are all leaves of one tree and the fruits of one branch."

Appendix

Books:

The Edgar Cayce Remedies by Dr. William McGarey 1983 Bantam Books

The Oil That Heals by Dr. William McGarey 1993 A.R.E. Press

The Miracle Oil by David Kukor 2008 A.R.E. Press

There is a River by Thomas Sugrue 1997 A.R.E.

Edgar Cayce: The Sleeping Prophet by Jess Stearn 1989 Bantam

Edgar Cayce Encyclopedia Of Healing by Reba Karp 1999 Grand Central Publishing

Web Sites:

www.edgarcayce.org

www.baar.com

www.heritagestore.com

www.facebook.com/edgarcayce

www.youtube.com/user/edgarcaycetv

Making A Castor Oil Pack   Using The Castor Oil Pack

Printed in the USA
CPSIA information can be obtained
at www.ICGtesting.com
LVHW080302300823
756710LV00019B/256

9 798452 529026